S0-AXW-655

DEC 1 5 2015

INFLUENZA 1918

INFLUENZA 1918

The Worst Epidemic in American History

Lynette Iezzoni

FOREWORD BY

David McCullough

Ventress Library
15 Library Plaza
Marshfield, MA 02050

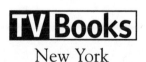

New York

DEC 1 5 2015

Copyright © 1999 TV Books, L.L.C.
All rights reserved. No part of this book may be reproduced in any form or by any means without permission in writing from the publishers, except by a reviewer who may quote brief passages in a review.

Influenza 1918 is the companion book to the television documentary "Influenza 1918" aired on PBS's documentary series *The American Experience*.

Publisher's Cataloging-in-Publication Data
Iezzoni, Lynette.
    Influenza 1918: the worst epidemic in American history / Lynette Iezzoni. — 1st ed.
      p. cm.
    Includes index.
    ISBN: 1-57500-108-X
    1. Influenza—History. 2. Epidemics—United States. I. Title.
    RC150.4.I39 1999
    614.5/18/0973   QBI99-135

Credits for photographs will be found on page 240.

The publisher has made every effort to secure permission to reproduce copyrighted material and would like to apologize should there have been any errors or omissions.

TV Books, L.L.C.
Publishers serving the television industry.
1619 Broadway, Ninth Floor
New York, NY 10019
www.tvbooks.com

Design by Joe Gannon and Rachel Reiss.

Manufactured in the United States.

Contents

The author would like to thank Ann Reid and
Jeffrey Taubenberger of the Armed Forces Institute of
Pathology for their help in deciphering the more obscure
aspects of the story's science. A great debt is owed
Ken Chowder, who wrote the film "Influenza 1918"
for *The American Experience,* and who provided
interview transcripts and other source materials.
The author would also like to thank Dr. Johan Hultin,
Mr. Michael Wind, Dr. Jody Balich, Kage Glantz,
and, for his patience and support, Robert Tomlinson.

Foreword

by David McCullough

In Boston the stock market closed. In Pennsylvania a statewide order shut down every place of amusement, every saloon. In Kentucky the Board of Health prohibited public gatherings of any kind, even funerals.

In 1918 America was caught up in the last horrific year of World War I. Yet the war had nothing to do with the extreme measures being taken. Deadly influenza, the so-called "Spanish flu," was sweeping the country, spreading terror everywhere.

The first documented deaths were in Boston. Explanations were offered, but in fact no one had an answer. Viruses were still largely unknown. But then to this day that particular flu virus is still one of the mysteries of the story.

Once started, the disease moved west in lethal waves that appeared to follow the lines of the railroads. The speed with which it killed was appalling, the loss of life unimaginable. By the time it had run its course in America, the epidemic took more than six hundred thousand lives.

It would be as if today, with our present population, more than 1.4 million people were to die in a sudden outbreak for which there was no explanation and no known cure.

It was said that every family lost someone. Certainly it seemed that way. I know my own family was no exception. Sarah Cowles, my great aunt—Sarah McCullough before she married—was one of fifty thousand cases in Pittsburgh, and one of the forty-five hundred who died there—in just one medium-sized city.

Could it happen again? Yes, indeed, which is part of the haunting power of this film.

We all hear and read a great deal about how wealthy we are as a nation. We're told our productivity is ahead of everybody else's, that more of our people are educated than any other nation's, that we live longer, have better retirement funds. But I wonder how often we stop to realize—and appreciate—how rich we Americans are in story.

This year, *The American Experience* is celebrating its tenth anniversary. In those ten years, over one hundred shows have been presented to audiences in the millions—an average of almost seven million viewers an episode. It is the country's only regularly scheduled historical documentary series, and what stories it can tell.

The American Experience brings to television the work of the best documentary filmmakers of our time, and in many cases their best work—David Grubin's "LBJ," Charles Guggenheim's "D-Day," Tom Lennon's "Battle of the Bulge," Austin Hoyt's "Carnegie," Ric Burns' "The Donner Party." *The American Experience* also brings to light stories about less well-known events and figures. Ed Gray and Janet Graham's marvelous "Orphan Trains" was scholarly groundbreaking, fine filmmaking that resulted in genuine historic discovery. Sam Pollard and Joyce Vaughn's powerful "Going Back to T-Town," about the race riots in Tulsa, Oklahoma, is another example of first-rate scholarship, investigation and interpretation. Again and again, the interviews done for our films, the research in archives and film and photograph collections, have turned up important new history, things of significance that have not been said or seen before.

Preface

We like to think of the past as a time of innocence. We were all children in the past, of course. Joy, sorrow, rage, and love came to us then in fierce waves of pure emotion undiluted with the complex sensibilities of the adult. Past and future held no sway; life was timeless: an eternal present. With a flick of our imagination, we could possess the power of Hercules, the magic of Merlin, the magnificence of Cleopatra.

Despite enormous proof to the contrary, we like to think of past civilizations as more innocent, less perilous than our own. After all, despite the lions of the Coliseum and the cruel despotism of Caligula, ancient Rome did not possess the atomic bomb. Despite bloody feuds between the kingdoms and the royal lords of Europe, despite the Inquisition and the Black Death, the Middle Ages did not occur beneath an earthly atmosphere of wispy, diminishing ozone. Like the arc of each individual life, civilizations experience their own life cycles, and with each cycle, each century, we seem to feel older, more encumbered, more grave.

We like to believe that America in the beginning of the twentieth century possessed an innocence, an optimism we have lost. While is true that America in 1918 possessed a certain innocence, it is also not true. True: in 1918 Henry Ford's frisky Model T rattled down America's burgeoning roads; coal production had given way to steel; skyscrapers were rising in New York, Boston, Cincinnati, and Los Angeles; and bridges were spanning the Hudson, the Mississippi, and San Francisco Bay. Electricity created a magical wonderland at Coney Island. The cinema amazed us, too, as did

9

airplanes, radios, ocean-liners. Change, progress, and excitement were in the air. Nevertheless, in small towns in America's heartland, life still ebbed and flowed with the seasonal rhythms of harvest and rest. Neighbors took care of neighbors. Doctors made house calls in horse and buggy, sometimes for the price of a chicken. Ours was the "Land of Milk and Honey," and in the past half century, we had beckoned welcome to millions and promised them a better life. As crowded ocean liners steamed towards Manhattan, scores of immigrants rode the heaving decks, searching the misty glare of New York Harbor for their first glimpse of Liberty Island and the Statue which represented the hope and promise of America. Millions thronged through America's gates, perfuming the land with exotic spices and filling her streets with the noise of concertinas, pushcart salesmen, and children's games. In bustling Philadelphia, Anna Milani was ten. Anna's family, parents and eleven children, shared a two-bedroom apartment, but Anna's memory, eighty years later, is of joy—a street filled with children, a street without fear, a street noisy with games...

> so many little games. We played tic tac toe, hop scotch, ring around the rosy. My brothers and sisters and I would sing songs—that was our style. My mother and father loved to sing as well. My father loved to sing opera and he would sing songs and we would follow him around. It was a happy, joyful life. We didn't have anything, but we had everything, because we were together.

Far from Anna Milani's Philadelphia, in Macon, Georgia, sugar magnolias and Spanish oaks lined broad, tranquil streets, and low rows of cotton and tobacco split the dusty red earth. Katharine Guyler was five. She recalls:

> Nineteen-eighteen was an age of innocence. My father was

my playmate, my best friend. He would take me out in his car and stop at the grocery store. The owner of the store would clap his hands and his men would come out in their white uniforms and he would say to them, "Miss Katherine is here. Go out and shake the Candy Tree, boys," and I would wait until they returned with little baskets full of candy. I must have known candy didn't grow in trees, but I wouldn't have given up the notion, because my father was enjoying it and I was enjoying it. Everyone was enjoying it.

Nineteen-eighteen was a time when anything—even candy trees—seemed possible. There was nothing Americans could not do.

We could even win the war that no one could win.

In April 1917, America had thrown her hat into the ring, entering the Great War on the side of the Allies. We had been stubbornly courted and we were full of ourselves: we had never lost a war. Patriotism gripped the nation. Liberty Loan rallies and parades drew thousands into the streets, and the most contemptuous word in America was "slacker." A hatred for all things German surged across the nation: the conductor Leopold Stokowski wrote President Woodrow Wilson to ask that Bach and Beethoven be dropped from all concert programs.

To seven-year-old Francis Russell, in Miss Sykes' third-grade class in Dorchester, Massachusetts, the Great War represented "the struggle of good against evil, light against darkness. For the victory of our boys, we ate peaches and baked the stones dry to be used for gas masks. One boy in Roxbury saved 2,000." The United States was a vigorous young nation, quickly becoming one of the greatest nations on Earth. With our peach pits and our doughboys, we would save Europe from catastrophe. With our "gasoline buggies," our washing machines, our electric mixers and our steel ingots, we would lead the world into the modern age.

Pride in America's prowess and ingenuity was matched by our newfound faith in science. In the late nineteenth century, Louis Pasteur and Robert Koch had ushered in the modern age of medicine, making the link between what could be glimpsed through a microscope (bacteria, germs) and infectious disease. For the first time, we could *see* what made us sick. We could isolate bacteria, create vaccines against them. From this, came triumph after medical triumph. In the mid-nineteenth century, one out of four children died before his second birthday. By 1918, as the result of pasteurization, the mortality rate among children had fallen dramatically. Researchers had developed vaccines for small pox, anthrax, rabies, diphtheria, and meningitis, cultured the bacteria responsible for tuberculosis, and made stunning progress in limiting the spread of insect-borne diseases like yellow fever and malaria. There seemed no limit to the knowledge of science, no limit to the power of the white-coated priests of medicine. Optimism abounded. America was the "can-do" country.

But looming within America were shadows which would soon envelop us. Despite our isolationist yearnings and the broad channels of the Atlantic and the Pacific, we were not as different or as isolated from the rest of the world as we liked to believe. Telephones, transoceanic telegraph cables, steam locomotives, automobiles and coal-powered steamships had created an increasingly interconnected, "shrinking" world, a world of flux and change. Empires were toppling, the age of kaisers, kings, and tsars expiring. In Europe and America, visual art was continuing its turbulent and dramatic metamorphosis: Cubism and Expressionism feeling the subversive touch of Dada. In the British Isles, James Joyce was penning *Ulysses*, Virginia Woolf, *Jacob's Room*; and T. S. Eliot was edging toward his modern epic poem, "The Wasteland." In Vienna, Sigmund Freud was weaving a tale of human psychological development which would forever change the way we think of our childhood, our parents, and our sexuality. And women on both sides of the Atlantic were demanding the vote. Agitations in the United States continued until 1920 when, with the nineteenth Amendment, American women joined their British sisters in winning the vote. Modernism—the new buzzword—demanded nothing less.

Most of all, the world of 1918 was a rapidly-industrializing world, a world of industrial strife. Mechanization of the work place—standardization, mass production, the assembly line— had spawned grimy, Dickensian work places, grueling sweatshops dominated by the thunder of machines, the fiery blasts of steel furnaces or the clank and rattle of bobbins and looms as thread was spun into cloth. Workers came into increasing conflict with management. In a tense, unstable Europe, industry turned to the machinery of war. The assassination of Archduke Franz Ferdinand, heir to the throne of Austria-Hungary, launched Europe into an explosive war—a war of nightmarish trenches, mustard gas, and staggering human losses, a war called by the British poet and soldier Robert Graves "the Sausage Machine."

In October 1917, the Bolsheviks seized power in Russia. Vladimir Lenin removed Russia from the European war. Proclaiming a "classless" society, Lenin urged workers throughout the world to "kick out kings and capitalists" and create a "dictatorship of the proletariat." Many were already restless. From Brooklyn to Madrid, Zurich to Argentina, Paris to West Virginia, workers were on strike: coal miners, postal workers, policemen, dock-workers, bank-clerks, railroad workers, garment workers, and boot and shoe workers. Violence—race riots, union strikes, anarchist bombings—was erupting all across America. Soon, the arrest of two obscure factory workers, Nicola Sacco and Bartolomeo Vanzetti, would culminate in one of the most celebrated and controversial murder trials of the century. Were Sacco and Vanzetti idealistic labor organizers or political extremists? America was divided.

Americans were divided about the war, too. Many families were still mourning losses from the Civil War. The European conflict was engrossing and exciting, but many Americans wondered why the assassination of an obscure Prussian Duke should cost American lives. In 1915, an anti-war protester set off a bomb in the U.S. Senate. As the violence escalated, Congress passed a law making "seditious" utterances a crime. Anyone who disagreed with U.S. war policy would be thrown into jail. A Vermont minister received a fifteen-year sentence for printing a pamphlet which called war "unchristian." In some states, it became illegal to teach German. In Washington D.C., an ambitious young FBI agent named J. Edgar Hoover, fearing America would follow the example of Bolshevik Russia, began compiling dossiers on suspected "radicals." Government "volunteers"—essentially, vigilantes—jailed some 20,000 suspected draft dodgers. In fact, protest against American involvement in World War I rivaled the furor a half-century later over Vietnam. Nevertheless, in an address to Congress on January 8, 1918, President Woodrow Wilson had outlined his "Fourteen Points" for achieving peace in Europe. America would lead the world into an age of freedom, democracy, and peace. We would still the turmoil in Europe, create a League of Nations.

Worlds removed from the bloody trenches of Europe, on a bustling street in South Philadelphia, Anna Milani and her brothers and sisters borrowed their father's trombone. They adorned a broom with a high hat and a picture of Kaiser Wilhelm, and marched out down the block. Trombone blaring, the Kaiser's hat teetering on the top of the broomstick, they led the neighborhood children in a rousing parade, singing: "Tramp, Tramp, Tramp, the Boys Are Marching. I Spy Kaiser at the Door. We'll get a lemon pie and we'll squash him in his eye and there won't be any Kaiser anymore." In Miss Sykes' class in Dorchester, Francis Russell was learning the Palmer Method of penmanship. In Macon, Georgia, Katharine Guyler had her Candy Tree.

At home, we felt safe.

Into this simple and complex world, onto this world stage stepped a ghostly, minuscule villain. Into this brash, changing world of Lenin and Freud, Picasso and Lillian Gish, King George V, Emperor Wilhelm II and Woodrow Wilson, stepped a player never seen before or since, a player who came and went entirely of her own volition, who even during her most savage acts never left the wings, never showed her face, never spoke. She penned her own script and acted it out in complete obscurity, in a realm too small for us to see or affect. She did not tell us her name, so we called her, like a character in a Dashiell Hammett mystery, "The Spanish Lady." But there was nothing Spanish or ladylike about her. Savage and capricious, wily as a coyote, she was a deft, avid traveler, and a swift, painful killer. In three waves, the three classic acts of a drama—an ominous flurry in the spring, devastation in the fall, and a brief reprise the next spring—she spread death from pole to pole. She was a microbe. An influenza virus. She caused the worst plague since the medieval Black Death, and by far the most catastrophic season of death in human history. In the end, over a billion people, more than half Earth's population, became sick. Between twenty-one and forty million perished. All in a few cruel, chaotic months.

This is a story of dying and forgetting, of bewilderment, chaos, bravery, and horror. This is a story of people who worked together and a country which almost fell apart, all in a single year in America. Yet this is a story no one knows and few remember. For as soon as the horror vanished from the face of the earth, the forgetting began.

Since the beginning of recorded history, waves of infectious disease have ravaged human populations, waxing and waning with mysterious, cyclical regularity. Even the name, influenza (from the Italian word for "influence"), speaks to the disease's inscrutable essence and timing. Over the centuries, influenza was called by many names: the "sweating sickness," the "jolly rant," "la grippe." From pathologic specimens collected during the 1889–90 "Russian flu" pandemic (a world-wide epidemic), Dr. Richard Pfeiffer, a Berlin microbiologist, isolated a bacteria which he and many others believed caused influenza: *Haemophilus influenzae*. In 1918, we had entered the modern age of medicine: the age of vaccines, pasteurization, sanitation, and insect control and we had identified "Pfeiffer's bacillus." How could influenza threaten us? Too, then (as now) we thought we knew the flu: a familiar, down-home malady which sent us to bed for three or four miserable days with fever, muscle aches, and congestion, then left us shaky for perhaps a week. It sickened millions, yet killed only the oldest and most feeble. As the old medical school saying went, influenza was a delightful disease. "Quite a Godsend! Everybody ill, nobody dying."

But the Spanish Lady was not the "flu," not any influenza we knew. In the words of historian Alfred Crosby, "Spanish influenza was a flu out of some sort of horror story. [It] turned people the color of wet ashes, drowned them in the fluids of their own bodies, and inspired names like the 'purple death.'" One moment a person was fine, the next incapacitated, delirious, dying. Wrenching coughs produced pints of greenish sputum. Blood gushed from the nose. Body temperature soared to 104 or 105 degrees. Oxygen-starved skin turned blue, purple, or deep mahogany brown. Massive pneumonia set in. In the end, patients literally drowned in their bloody, fluid-filled lungs. It was a savage, swift, terrifying death. And Spanish influenza tended to kill exactly the people the flu usually spared. The highest number of deaths occurred among people between fifteen and forty years of age, robust young people in the prime of life.

In the autumn of 1918, Spanish influenza exploded across America, quickly engulfing the nation in plague. The epidemic became a public-health crisis like none before or since. The illness baffled medical science at every turn. Things were upside down and backwards. Influenza was not supposed kill in such numbers, kill so violently, or kill the healthy and the young. Dozens of different vaccines were pumped into hundreds of thousands of arms. None worked. The panicked, bewildered public turned to folk cures: wearing necklaces of chicken feathers, keeping an ace of diamonds in a shoe, inhaling the acrid smoke of burning corncobs, chanting voodoo spells. After a century of stunning progress, the rising authority of medical science vanished in a matter of a few horrific weeks.

In September 1918, 12,000 Americans died of influenza. In October, 195,000 died. As the death toll mounted, the rich tapestry of American life began to unravel.

During seventeen horrifying, apocalyptic weeks, Spanish influenza sickened some twenty-five million Americans. An estimated 670,000 died. The Spanish Lady killed more Americans than have been killed in all the wars of the twentieth century combined. Yet we seem to have forgotten her. Why should America's most catastrophic season of death, one which happened a mere eighty years ago, be stricken from our collective consciousness? Critic and author, H. L. Mencken lived through the pandemic. Writing in 1956, he mused,

> The epidemic is seldom mentioned and most Americans have apparently forgotten it. This is not surprising. The human mind always tries to expunge the intolerable from memory.

Of course, many never forgot. For those who lived through the horror, for those lucky enough to survive, adults and children alike, this was the moment when life changed irrevocably. Innocence was lost. For many Americans, the autumn of 1918 became the moment which separated "before" from "after," the moment when "once upon a time" became that time a week, a day, an hour ago—the time before the flu. Officials in the Northeast sent urgent warnings to the West: "Hunt up your wood-workers and set them to making coffins. Then take your street laborers and set them to digging graves." But in 1918, America ran out of coffins. America ran out of gravediggers. The nation's promise failed. For this time, America did not recognize itself, and perhaps that is why we have chosen to forget.

In July 1996, Dr. Amy Krafft, a molecular biologist at the Armed Forces Institute of Pathology in Washington, D.C., carefully extracted a minute scrap of lung from a small paraffin mold. The lung had been preserved at the National Tissue Repository, a sprawling Army morgue housing more than 2.5 million autopsy specimens dating back to the time of the Civil War. Krafft is part of a team of molecular biologists specializing in the sophisticated and arcane business of recovering viruses from severely decomposed tissue or long-preserved pathologic specimens. They are, in effect, viral archaeologists. The scrap of lung which held Krafft's interest belonged to a twenty-one-year-old soldier who died of Spanish influenza at Fort Jackson, South Carolina, on September 26, 1918—Private Roscoe Vaughn.

In the 1950s, with the invention of the electron microscope, scientists glimpsed viruses for the first time. Still, no one had ever seen the Spanish Lady. Influenza viruses change constantly, and she had long since mutated beyond recognition, taking her secrets with her to countless millions of graves all over the world. Attempts to recover traces of Spanish influenza from flu victims buried in the natural freezer of Alaska's permafrost had failed. Influenza viruses are infinitely delicate. They begin breaking down the moment a person dies. But the techniques of molecular biology were becoming ever more ingenious. In the A.F.I.P. lab, even a *dead* virus could be coaxed to yield up her secrets.

In July 1996, nearly eighty years after Spanish influenza engulfed the world in plague, the virus was seen for the first time. From the fragile remnants of virus recovered from Private Roscoe Vaughn's lung, scientists have begun unlocking the secrets of this savage and elusive killer.

Only one thing is certain. What became a global catastrophe, claiming millions of human lives, began with a small and random act of nature. In all likelihood, the "Spanish Lady" was born in America's heartland. Kansas. Her creation story seems as quaint and harmless as a fairy tale.

A bird, probably a wild duck, rose from a lake in Canada. Flying south towards its winter nesting ground, the duck passed over Kansas. The duck sojourned, or perhaps simply defecated, in a pond. Perhaps a pig was wallowing in the pond. Perhaps children were playing there. A chance encounter occurred. Perhaps between a duck and a pig. Perhaps between a duck and a man, woman, or child. Perhaps between a pig and a man. Most probably between all three. From this, a virus was spawned, a submicroscopic creature which, with all the innocence and cunning of nature herself, created the incalculable human tragedy of Influenza 1918.

Chapter 1

Spring 1918: Kansas

The beginning came with an ill wind in Kansas. One day in the early spring of 1918, soldiers at Fort Riley, Kansas, burned tons of horse manure. A gale kicked up, and a choking dust storm swept over the prairie—a stinking yellow haze which stymied trucks on the Golden Belt Highway and stopped Union Pacific trains dead in their tracks. The sky went black in Kansas. All across Fort Riley, a sprawling, crowded camp of twenty-six thousand, soldiers raced for cover. Drafty barracks creaked in the howling wind. Grit sifted through knotholes and cracks. For three hours, the storm raged. Then suddenly the fierce winds died. A ghostly sun, haloed with dust, slowly regained her strength. Her diaphanous light revealed the filthy debris of a prairie dust storm. Fort Riley's twenty thousand acres were completely covered in a dense shroud of dirt and ash. Ordered from their barracks, given buckets and brooms, soldiers began cleaning up the mess. They toiled long past midnight, sweeping, raking, shoveling, and coughing.

Fifty years earlier, General George Armstrong Custer and his 7th Cavalry had thundered across these Kansas badlands. Like other remote forts out of the American Wild West, Fort Riley provided a haven for emigrants spilling west into the Indian territories, the home of the Apache, the Comanche, the Sioux. During three decades of bloody Indian Wars, Fort Riley housed the U.S. Army in austere, spartan style. In 1918, the din of covered wagons and the pop of Winchesters, Spencer Carbines, and Colt revolvers had been replaced by the rumble of trucks on the Golden Belt Highway and the squeal of trolleys linking Fort Riley and its sprawling subdivision Camp Funston with neighboring Manhattan and Junction City. What had not changed was the clip-clop and whinny of horses. Thousands of horses and mules were attached to the army's cavalry and maintenance divisions, animals which produced nine thousand tons of manure each month. Mule skinners had no choice but to burn it. Night and day, manure smoldered, sending dark plumes of acrid smoke into the broad Kansas sky.

Eleven months had passed since America had entered the European War. Since then, her peacetime army had swelled from 190,000 men to more than two million. Rampant overcrowding in the nation's bases worried U.S. Surgeon General William C. Gorgas. Early in 1918, testifying before the Senate Military Affairs Committee, Gorgas warned that widespread overcrowding was creating conditions ripe for the spread of infectious disease. A grizzled, white-haired veteran of the fight against yellow fever, Gorgas understood the threat posed by life's most common hazards: mosquitoes, spoiled food, pooling sewage. He urged that mobilization of the Armed Forces be delayed for two to three months until better facilities could be constructed. Back in Kansas, Fort Riley's chief medical officer, Colonel Edward R. Schreiner, shared Gorgas' concern. A sober, forty-five-year-old surgeon, Schreiner presided over the camp's 3,068-bed hospital. Fort Riley's hastily-assembled barracks, crowded with the swelling ranks of Midwestern inductees, were little better than the spartan quarters which had housed weary soldiers during the previous century's Indian Wars. Most barracks lacked heat, hot water, and even latrines. Drafty and uninsulated, they offered scant protection against winter's icy blizzards, frenzied prairie dust storms, and the sweltering heat of July and August, when temperatures soared to 107 degrees. Schreiner's hospital, an amalgam of old limestone, brick, and clapboard buildings, was a weathered veteran of the Spanish-American War. Daily quarantine flags, run up the flagpole, announced outbreaks of pneumonia, measles, grippe, mumps, and spinal meningitis.

On Monday March 11, 1918—two days after the foul, dusty squall which had enveloped Fort Riley—Private Albert Gitchell, a cook, reported to the camp hospital before breakfast. He had a fever, sore throat, headache. Just the flu. Nothing to worry about. A minute later, however, another sick soldier showed up. Then another. By noon, the baffled hospital staff had 107 cases on their hands. By week's end: 522. In the next month, they saw well over a thousand.

One of those was Private John Lewis Barkley. Barkley was eighteen years old, from Holden, Missouri. A shy loner with an embarrassing stutter, Barkley had spent his childhood roaming the Missouri woods hunting rabbits, deer, and quail, emulating his hero, Daniel Boone. The call to arms had captured Barkley's imagination. He would become an army scout, creeping through the woods of France behind enemy lines. Fort Riley, however, was proving far different from Barkley's romantic Europe, and no part of Fort Riley was more dismal than the influenza ward of Schreiner's hospital. One night, Barkley was awakened by an icy hand gripping his arm. The soldier in the next bed was delirious with fever. He mumbled, thrashed. Blood streamed from his nose. The soldier dug his fingers into Barkley's arm. Then he died.

A total of forty-eight soldiers died of influenza at Fort Riley that spring. In each case, the cause of death was listed as pneumonia. Colonel Schreiner was disconcerted. Why should so many healthy young men develop massive, secondary pneumonia and die from "flu"? In many cases, the symptoms were highly unusual, even horrifying: labored breathing, violent coughs, projectile nosebleeds. Faces turned a ghostly blue. Bodily functions, includ-

ing the heart, became depressed—a paradoxical finding in a setting of high fever. Patients literally drowned in their bloody, fluid-
filled lungs. And it all happened quickly. Young men went from
robust health to death in a matter of days, sometimes only hours.

In cultures taken from his patients, Schreiner found evidence
of *Haemophilus influenzae*, Pfeiffer's bacillus, the hemophilic
(blood-nourished) bacteria widely believed to be the cause of influenza. Cultures also revealed a host of other bacteria. Had Pfeiffer's bacillus *caused* this strange, deadly flu? Or was *Haemophilus
influenzae* merely an incidental finding?

And then the dying stopped. Most of the sick got better. Fort
Riley's outbreak of "pneumonia" ended, vanishing just as mysteriously as it came.

In Goldsboro, North Carolina, wagons rumbled into town
every Saturday, converging on Main Street alongside the railroad
tracks. The sluggish rhythms of small town life quickened. Farmers unloaded bushels of produce: collards, peaches, tomatoes,
corn. Other vendors crowded in, too. Children scampered among
the carts. Dan Tonkel, the son of a Goldsboro clothing merchant,
was one of those children. In 1918, he was seven. Dan remembers:

> The farmers would park their wagons on the railroad tracks,
> because the trains didn't run on Saturdays. They sold all kinds
> of produce and other people sold chickens and some vendors
> sold things like snake oil and rheumatism liniment. I remem-
> ber there was a snake oil salesman who always brought a rattle
> snake with him. He let the snake crawl all over him while he
> sold his oil. He said the oil had come from this snake and it
> would cure all our ills.

But Dan Tonkel had few ills. Life for Dan was peaceful, simple, and predictable. School, chores, and helping his father in the store, watching him buy and sell. Saturdays, however, brought the excitement of the farmers' market. Then, Dan's father would take the family to a movie at Goldsboro's theater and buy everyone an ice cream.

> All week I looked forward to that ice cream. Ice cream cones were five cents in those days, and if I could earn a nickel here or there, I could buy myself an ice cream during the week. My uncle Benny would give me a nickel for heating up the water for his bath and scrubbing his back in the bathtub. And a saleslady at my father's store, Miss Leah, sometimes slipped me a nickel as well. Miss Leah used to show me how to do everything you could do in the yard goods department. She would roll off a yardage of cloth and say, "Come here, Daniel, you cut the fabric." She'd give me her scissors and let me cut the fabric. She and I were very close. I was her pet and once in a while, she'd slip me a nickel for that ice cream cone I so wanted. She was bribing me, of course—but I loved her for it. We had a gentle, peaceful time, Miss Leah and I. Life was simple in Goldsboro, life was very peaceful.

In March 1918, a thousand workers at the Ford Motor Company in Detroit came down with influenza. During April and May, five hundred of San Quentin Prison's nineteen hundred inmates became sick with flu; three died. Outbreaks of influenza occurred at army camps in California, Florida, Virginia, Alabama, South Carolina, and Georgia. Surgeon General William Gorgas reported epidemic influenza at Camps Oglethorpe, Gordon, Grant, Lewis, Doniphan, Fremont, Sherman, Logan, Hancock, Kearney, McClellan, and others. Odd, but no one was much alarmed. Microbes had always wreaked havoc in the crowded quarters of war. In all previous wars, disease had proved more deadly than any combination of arrows, bullets, cannons, and bayonets. Although vaccines and other medicines, improved sanitation, and strict codes of cleanliness had dramatically re-duced outbreaks of insect-, water-, and food-borne diseases (dis-eases which had plagued armies as recently as the Civil War and the Spanish-American War), air-borne diseases continued to thrive in the military. Still, epidemics were to be expected in the camps of war. And the U.S. military was pushing hard to get troops to France, where General John J. "Black Jack" Pershing was planning the first American offensive.

By April, influenza, following the trail of soldiers amassing and moving throughout the nation, had spread to most cities in America. But this spring "wave" passed nearly unnoticed. Bul-letins from Surgeon General Gorgas revealing epidemic out-breaks of influenza in the Armed Forces were not matched by civilian reports, because such civilian reports simply did not exist. The United States did not have an effective, established system of federal, state, and local public health authorities; the Commissioner of Health for the state of Washington explained the inefficiency of his organization by saying his staff was paid very little, "and their policy is to do as much as the pay justifies." Later review of death certificates from the nation's fifty largest cities revealed widespread influenza among the civilian popula-tion in March and April, but the 1918 volumes of *The Journal of the American Medical Association* made no mention of this. Most state health departments did not even ask for influenza to be re-ported—it was not considered serious enough. Too, influenza was often an ambiguous diagnosis. Just what *was* the flu? How did in-fluenza differ from a bad cold? If influenza resulted in pneumonia, and the pneumonia proved fatal, had the victim died of influenza or pneumonia? Bacterial analyses of the sputum of flu patients re-vealed a veritable pea-soup of microbes: Pfeiffer's bacillus, pneu-mococci, streptococci, and many others. Just what (if anything)

did this mean? What *microbe* verified the diagnosis of influenza?
Statistical or epidemiological evidence of a flu epidemic was also
obscured by the fact that, when influenza proved fatal, the cause
of death was usually recorded as pneumonia. In 1918, before the
development of sulfa drugs and penicillin, pneumonia was an ex-
tremely common form of death. Little could be done for the patient suffering pneumonia except, as the homily went, "Put him
to bed with a pot of tea and honey, and God Bless."

This "spring wave" of influenza barely affected America's mortality rates. Still, the disease displayed ominous features. Autopsies revealed widespread bloody hemorrhage and swelling of the
lungs. And oddly, this flu was killing young, healthy people. Mortality statistics drawn from army sources and death certificates in
New York City; Minneapolis; San Francisco; Seattle; Lowell,
Massachusetts; and Birmingham, Alabama, showed a "spike"
among twenty-one to twenty-nine-year-olds. The people who influenza usually spared were dying of this flu.

In the nation at large, no one gave these strange little spates
of death another thought. Nineteen-eighteen was a momentous
year for a nation just edging into modern times. Most families,
like Dan Tonkel's, still relied on outdoor toilets and kerosene
lamps, but the newfangled gadgets of modern life began rolling
into homes: the typewriter, the hand-cranked phonograph, the
washing machine. In 1913, the first home refrigerator had gone
on sale in Chicago. In 1914, red and green traffic lights had
flashed for the first time in Cleveland, Ohio. In 1915, Alexander
Graham Bell (in New York) and Thomas A. Watson (in San
Francisco) had conducted the first transcontinental telephone
call. From Pyrex dishware to the classification of the four major
blood groups, from the heating pad to Hans Geiger's radiation
detector for alpha particles, from windshield wipers to the iden-

tification of chromosomes as carriers of heredity, new discoveries and inventions were rocking the world. And nothing more so than the automobile. The loud vroom of "gasoline-buggies" was heard throughout the land. Henry Ford's "Tin Lizzie" was joined by the Marmon, the Kisselkar, and the Paige-Detroit.

Katherine Guyler's father was one of the first drivers in Macon, Georgia. She recalls:

> Everybody wanted to take a ride. I mean, you just plain needed to take a ride. There were no paved roads in Macon, so the car was always getting stuck. But whenever that happened, a neighbor would just send over a mule to pull the car out of the mud. Macon was like that. Macon was a chummy kind of a place.

In 1918, William Maxwell was growing up in Lincoln, Illinois, a modest Midwestern town of twelve thousand. Cars had appeared in Lincoln, too. William Maxwell's grandfather had purchased an automobile, "full of leather straps and brass headlights. It was sort of half carriage, half car, and it sat like a monument in front of his house."

When William was six, his father bought their family a car.

> Our carriage horse had a tendency to buck and run away, and it made my mother nervous. So my father sold the horse, tore down the barn, built a garage, and we moved into the modern age with a seven passenger Buick. The car got about six miles to the gallon, and had a tendency to stall on hills. On the other hand, it was enormous and there was room in the back seat for my mother and her best friend and her best friend's little girl. The little girl and I would lie on the floor at our mothers' feet comfortably, there was so much room. Illinois was very hot in the summer, so it was a great pleasure to drive out into the country to cool off. Every Sunday, we would take the Buick

for a spin in the country. Of course, Sunday was God's day in Lincoln; there were more churches in town than I could count on my two hands. But my father had had enough of church-going, so on Sundays we'd take the Buick out into the country... go fishing and have a picnic.

Like Katherine Guyler's Macon, William Maxwell's Lincoln, Illinois, was a town straight out of America's heartland, a town which will, as such, always remain deeply embedded in America's nostalgic imagination. In 1918, the family of Michael Donohue lived in a community which was just as much a sign of the times, just as integral to the nation's changing mood. No sugar magnolias bloomed in the Donohues' Philadelphia. No swings creaked on broad verandahs. Fire wagons raced through crowded streets, dragged by galloping horses. Pushcarts rattled, accompanied by bellowing shouts and entreaties. Songs were sung, arguments were had, gossip was relayed, prayers were murmured in a dozen languages. America's cities were flooded with immigrants. Irish, Italians, Poles, Germans, Chinese, and scores of others crowded into bustling neighborhoods, slums usually— friendly, argumentative ghettos perfumed with the odor of jerked meat and piquant spices and the smoky, intransigent pollution of coal fires. In labyrinthine alleys, wash fluttered on tangled clotheslines. Inside dim, Gothic-style churches, votives simmered beneath terra-cotta martyrs. Clouds of incense swelled and dissipated. Baptisms, weddings, and funerals evoked the sounds and smells of the "Old Country."

In an Irish enclave in West Philadelphia, Michael Donohue's great-grandfather owned a small, neighborhood funeral home. In 1918, he had just purchased a motorized hearse.

It was one of the first motorized hearses in Philadelphia. Before that, our hearse had always been drawn by horses. That

car was my great-grandfather's pride and joy. He was so proud
of it he even had pictures taken. It had our family name—
Donohue—engraved on the side.

Cars were changing the road map, the routines of America.
War was changing America, too. Americans were "hooveriz-
ing": as Food Controller Herbert Hoover preached, they were
observing the "gospel of the clean plate." And thousands of
young men were leaving towns like Philadelphia, Lincoln, and
Macon for army camps and the battlefields of Europe. In theaters across the nation, *The Kaiser, the Beast of Berlin* played to
packed houses. Newspaper headlines screamed: "Huns Live in
Terror of Yankee Divisions." War eclipsed nearly everything.
Even children thought of little else.

Francis Russell was seven years old, attending the Martha
Baker School in Dorchester, a section of Boston. He later wrote:

> That was the stupendous and embracing fact, even to us in
> Miss Sykes's third-grade room, the war to end wars, to make
> the world safe for democracy. Like the wicked stepmother or
> the witch of the fairy tales, the Germans, the Huns, with their
> lustful Kaiser Bill and the ridiculous Clown Prince would meet
> the fate of all dark spirits, witches, and wicked stepmothers.
>
> "Beat the Hun!" Those barbarians we were fighting had
> started it all by attacking brave little Belgium and torturing
> women and children there—the poor suffering Belgians, most
> crucified of people. "Beat the Hun!" The Third Liberty Loan
> poster showed a porcine German with heavy carnal mustache
> and spiked helmet silhouetted against the background of a
> flaming town as he dragged a trembling, long-haired girl with
> him toward the shadows.

For Francis Russell, there would be no frosting on birthday

cakes until the grand struggle with "lustful Bill" ended. Until the Allies claimed victory, there was the Junior Red Cross to join; there were pennies to be saved for Thrift Stamps.

> We joined the Junior Red Cross and wore the rectangular cel-luloid pins in our button-holes. Then there were the Thrift Stamps at twenty-five cents each for us to buy from Mr. Gib-ney the postman. Mr. Gibney gave us a little book to paste the stamps in. Each space to be filled had a motto like "A Penny Saved is a Penny Earned" or "Great Oaks from Little Acorns Grow." When we had twenty stamps we exchanged them with Mr. Gibney for a War-Savings Certificate. Instead of sugar we used Karo Corn Syrup. The red Karo cans had yellow syrup and the blue ones white. Neither tasted very good, and there was no frosting any more even for birthday cakes, because the sugar had to go to the starving Belgians.

Across the nation, communities mobilized to serve nearby army bases. The soldier was the darling of America and neighbors pitched in to help "our boys." Once a week, William Maxwell's mother volunteered with the war effort. He remembers:

> She would put on a white dress, and wrap a dishtowel around her head with a red cross on it. She rolled bandages mostly. In school, we saved prune pits which were supposed to be turned into gas masks. I don't know how many gas masks were made from prune pits, but I shouldn't think very many. In any event, it gave us a sense of helping with the war.

But even communities which threw open their doors to Amer-ica's "darlings" were not without ambivalence. Wariness re-mained about the war, the sudden influx of strangers, and the army's confiscation of local land and resources.

Just outside Macon, Georgia, Camp Wheeler was swelling with recruits. Katherine Guyler recalls:

> It was an invasion, you see. People in Macon didn't greet the soldiers with all that much excitement, because we didn't know who they were. Also, there was a great difference in opinion about whether or not we should even be in the European war. Many families had not recovered from the Civil War. People in Macon wondered: "Why are we giving up all this land, turning it over to the army for a war in Europe? And Camp Wheeler is just messing up the whole community, with all the soldiers coming in—and the patriotic things you have to do, like stop eating sugar." These were very important issues to families. I remember my mother made fudge with some sugar she'd been hoarding, so if anyone visited they wouldn't see any sugar, just a little fudge. In those days, women had big families and big jobs to do. They weren't free to volunteer, other than what they always did, neighbors helping neighbors. But there was a patriotic feeling and it was growing larger. Soon, all the women worked with soldiers. It became a patriotic duty and people found time to do it. We all lived rather dull lives and the war was exciting.

But the war was not going well. When Bolshevik Russia dropped out of the war, Germany had shunted troops west, achieving numerical superiority. From October 24 to November 12, 1917, the armies of the Central Powers had advanced into Italy, devastating the Italian Second Army at Caporetto (costing the Italians six hundred thousand casualties and prisoners), and handing the Allies a grave defeat. Warily, the French and English waited. "A terrible blow is imminent," French Premier Georges Clemenceau said in March 1918. "Tell your Americans to come quickly." General Pershing, commander of the American Expeditionary Force (A.E.F.), cabled the War Department. He needed four million soldiers to win. Bring on more doughboys.

On March 21, 1918, the German offensive began. The Kaiser's troops quickly overran 1,250 square miles of France and began shelling Paris. For 140 days, "Big Bertha" howitzers rained down shells on Paris. If the Germans could drive a wedge between the French and British, they could force the British back across the Channel and achieve victory. The Allies were outnumbered, with 173 divisions to Germany's 192. Only one choice remained: hang on until the Americans arrived.

And the doughboys were coming. That summer and fall, 1.5 million American soldiers crossed the ocean for war.

Some came from Kansas. Loaded onto troop trains, they were packed into ships "like salt cod in a keg." The conditions were absolutely perfect for the spread of infectious disease. The symbiosis of war and flu, the two great engines of death, had begun. In the end, the soldiers would bring far more death with their microbes than with their guns.

It was a calm summer. Still, in one town, a doctor noted that all his prize roses suddenly wilted. In another, a huge flock of owls came out of nowhere and hooted eerily from every windowsill. In still another, a sailor swore that a statue of the Virgin shed a tear. In Montreal, a cloudless sky grew black as pitch; a fortune teller predicted a time of great pestilence. People opened their Bibles: "Let all the inhabitants of the land tremble; for the day of the Lord cometh, a day of clouds and thick darkness...nothing shall escape. The people shall be much pained: all faces shall gather blackness."

Pentecostal ministers paid a visit to Brooklyn Street in Philadelphia. The preachers stood on the corner of Brooklyn and Fairmont Streets and passionately predicted an imminent calamity. Harriet Ferrell, who lived at 703 Brooklyn Street, remembers:

People gathered, but they more or less ignored the preachers. People thought they were Christian enough...nothing bad would happen to them. They didn't think they needed sermons, especially street sermons. So the Pentecostal ministers did what was done in Biblical days. They shook the dust from their sandals and prophesied: "Soon you will experience a terrible calamity. After that we will return and you will be very interested in what we have to say."

In Goldsboro, North Carolina, Dan Tonkel raced down a dusty road on his bicycle. He skidded to a stop. The sweltering heat created an illusion of silvery lakes on the road, like pools of liquid mercury. Still, Dan thought he had seen something. There, just at the edge of the scrub pines, was a twenty dollar bill. Dan brought it home and gave it to his father. His father said, "This will go towards Aunt Tilly's surgical bill."

My aunt Tilly had just had an appendectomy. She was in the hospital and the surgery bill was $50.00. I recall that because it seemed like so much to pay a doctor.

Fees were nominal in those days. Two or three dollars, maybe. I don't think a doctor ever charged as much as five dollars, unless perhaps they did some surgery. Doctors were full of humility. There was no such thing as going to an office or making an appointment. You would just send a child up to the doctor's house to say, "Hey, Doc, my little brother's sick or my mother's sick, please come over." And he would come over with his little satchel and do what he thought best. He always took your temperature; he'd put a thermometer under your tongue, feel your pulse, and take your blood pressure. From that point on, it was pretty much hit and miss. Doctors had very little to offer. A few vaccines, a few little pills, morphine. If he didn't have the cure-all in his little black satchel, there was little else he could do. Fees were very low and people were not in a hurry to pay. They'd say, "Oh, Doc, I'll pay you later." Lots of people paid with a system of bartering. I remember one of our neighbors saying, "Well, I've got to go get a couple of chickens and take 'em up to the doctor, because I owe him two dollars and I'd better give him something to keep him happy." I think the worst I ever had done to me was having a boil lanced. Children were always getting boils in those days because we ran around barefoot in the dirt.

In a dilapidated Army Hospital in Cittadella, Italy, Second Lieutenant Giuseppe Agostoni huddled over a dying soldier. A twenty-five-year-old medic, Agostoni had watched in horror as influenza ravaged his regiment. But what kind of flu was this? Men were choking to death, gagging on the bloody regurgitations of their fluid-filled lungs. Faces turned grey, purple, then brown. Labored breathing produced a weird, duck-like quack. Agostoni rummaged through his bag for a 23 cc. syringe. Perhaps draining some of the bloody fluid would help relieve the soldier's congestion. Agostoni stuck the soldier's arm. He slowly pulled back on the syringe, but the blood clotted. After only 10 cc., the syringe failed. The blood of the dying soldier was black and gummy, as viscous as tar.

All across Europe, soldiers and civilians alike were down with a strangely savage flu.

The earliest reports of epidemic influenza had come in mid-April 1918, among the American Expeditionary Force disembarking at the French port of Bordeaux. By May, Americans were down with "three day fever," the French suffering from "la grippe," the Germans, "Flanders Fever" or "Blitzkatarrh," and the Italians, "sandfly fever." In Spain, eight million people were ill, including one third of all the residents of Madrid. Spain's King Alfonso XIII fell sick. So did Britain's King George V. In Berlin,

Kaiser Wilhelm and 160,000 fellow Berliners were ill. All across Europe, trams stopped running and businesses and government offices closed. Influenza began affecting the schedules of war. For twelve days in May, the British Grand Fleet remained docked; 10,313 British sailors were sick. During three days in June, P.U.O. (Pyrexia of Unknown Origin) sent three thousand British soldiers to hospital in Etaples, France; at British G.H.Q., seven hundred were sick. On the other side of the Hindenburg Line, Germans were failing at their posts as well. Some flu-ravaged divisions were down to fifty men. The commander of the German forces, General Erich von Ludendorff, complained: "It was a grievous business, having to listen every morning to the Chiefs of Staff's recital of the number of influenza cases, and their complaints about the weakness of their troops." Ludendorff later blamed the failure of Germany's July offense (which nearly resulted in German victory) on the reduced strength and morale of his troops, due, in part, to influenza.

The pain began behind the eyes, spread to the ears, the neck, the spine, and the legs. A soaring fever, chills, and delirium made for a painful, mind-numbing ordeal. In some cases, after three or four miserable days the malady began to subside. But other patients developed massive pneumonia and death came swiftly. "Purulent bronchitis"? "Flanders Fieber"? The grippe?

By now, most Europeans were calling the illness Spanish influenza.

In February, influenza had affected San Sebastian, a seaside town on the northern coast of Spain. Town officials, worried about a loss of summer tourism, tried to contain news of the outbreak. A prison in Almeria, on Spain's southern coast, also experienced a severe outbreak of flu. Again, officials tried to suppress reports of the illness. But as winter eased into spring, influenza spread through Spain, and King Alfonso's illness made headlines in *El Sol*, San Sebastian's malady and the epidemic among Almeria's convicts were remembered. Unlike the combatant nations of Europe, nonbelligerent Spain had no wartime censorship of the press, no propaganda network to suppress news of epidemic disease among citizenry or soldiers. Soon Spain had joined the venerable ranks of nations whose names were attached to pandemics, a venerable (if often unjust) tradition dating back to 1510. The Spanish government formed a medical commission which concluded that the scourge bearing its country's name had originated in Turkestan, Russia. Russia was unconvinced. As influenza struck the city of Murom, *Pravda* announced: "*Ispanka* [the Spanish Lady] is in town."

Germany's General Ludendorff commenced the first of his five massive summer offenses. In each, the Germans gained ground, but none—including the last, the thunderous "Second Battle of the Marne"—proved decisive. The Allied commander, French Marshal Ferdinand Foch, sensed a changing tide. Since March, half a million German soldiers had died. The Allies had lost slightly more, but were being replenished with three hundred thousand Americans each month. Foch counterattacked at Château Therry. On August 8, he surprised the Germans at the Somme. Between August 8 and 12, twenty thousand German soldiers were killed and twenty-one thousand taken prisoner. Ludendorff later referred to August 8 as Germany's "Black Day." Indeed, the fortunes of war were changing. But U.S. Army medics, surgeons, and nurses, overwhelmed with the bloody human debris of battle, had little to celebrate. Nor did they have time to inquire into the peculiarities of "Spanish influenza."

One soldier who had never forgotten his terrifying encounter with influenza was Private John Lewis Barkley. For eight months, Barkley had crept through the woods of Troyes, Rozay, Belleville, and Château Thierry, smeared in wet clay and dressed in a bulky burlap sack camouflaged with leaves, relaying back information on German troop movements to U.S. Army Headquarters (H.Q.)

by field telephone and Morse code. With him were his two
Cherokee Indian buddies: Floyd and "Jesse" James. The three had
met while desperately sick in the influenza ward of a hospital in
Fort Riley, Kansas. When they recovered, they swore an oath to
stick together, take care of each other, and never again enter a
hospital. Although Barkley had been bayoneted in the chest,
"Jesse" had sniffed mustard gas, and Floyd was nursing a bullet
wound in his left arm, they had eschewed medics and patched
each other up with iodine and bandages. On the eve of the battle at St. Mihiel, the three reaffirmed their oath: "No pill-roller
is going to put a toe-tag on us."

During the summer months, Spanish influenza ebbed and
flowed across the smoldering battlefields and ancient provinces
of Europe. In July, just as the combatant armies were experiencing some relief, flu surged through the civilian population. Europeans were wearily enduring their fifth year of war. Food,
clothing, soap, coal, and other essentials were in short supply or
virtually unattainable. Leather ripped from the seats of trains
was made into shoes. Women substituted beet-juice for non-
existent rouge. In the window of Cartier's, Paris, a shimmering
diamond necklace adorned a single precious nugget of coal. In
Italy, wedding rings were being sold for sausage. In London, signs
reading "Eat Less Bread—Let the Menu Beat the U-Men" were
ubiquitous. In Cologne, Germany, thousands were, in the words
of Mayor Konrad Adenauer, "too exhausted to hate." During the
summer of 1918, thousands fell sick with influenza in London,
Hamburg, Paris, and Copenhagen—fifty-three thousand in tiny
Switzerland alone. In cities already depleted of young, draft-age
men, nearly half of those who died were between the ages of
twenty and forty-five, society's most robust, productive members. Omnipresent but denied, censored, or under-reported, lost
amid the carnage and drama of war, the Spanish Lady moved
north, south, east, and west. Traveling on ships, trucks, and

trains, she crossed oceans, deserts, and mountain ranges, making her way into Scandinavia, Greece, Egypt, West Africa, Russia, India, China, Japan, and South America.

In four months, the microbe rounded the globe. In this, her "spring wave," she had already killed tens of thousands. But during the summer of 1918, she was oddly absent from the United States. For most of that summer, America was statistically healthier than it had ever been. Still, in crowded army camps, hundreds of thousands of recruits were being readied for the trenches of Europe. In these camps, hospitals were being hurriedly constructed, built with less thought, a physician later remarked, than a farmer would give to the planning of milk barns. Packed onto crowded trains, routed to embarkation ports in the east, troops were sardined into the airless hulls of steel battleships. In June, 279,000 American soldiers sailed for Europe, in July, 300,000, and in August, 286,000. In the last six months of the war, 1.5 million American soldiers landed in Europe.

The world was restless. All kinds of vessels were crossing the world's oceans. The movement, merging, mingling of peoples was unprecedented. Ships from New Zealand, re-coaling in Sierra Leone, encountered British ships heading to South Africa, India, and Australia. Allied vessels, hoping to attack Germany from the rear, were slipping into the White Sea, down the wilds of the Dvina River, to the Russian city of Archangel. Five hundred multinational men-of-war were anchored in the French port of Brest; 791,000 doughboys were pouring through Brest's *Depôt de la Marine* and meeting up with flu-ridden French divisions. Influenza was everywhere, borne invisibly, on breath. In Freetown, Sierra Leone, five hundred of the Sierra Leone Coaling Company's six hundred colliers fell sick with influenza. Archangel and all of embattled Russia was engulfed in flu. Influenza-ridden ships were arriving in American ports. The *City of Exeter* limped into Philadelphia from Liverpool; twenty-eight crew members were dispatched immediately to hospitals. An Indian vessel, *Somali*, deposited eighty-nine influenza victims on Grosse Isle in the Gulf of Saint Lawrence. On August 12, the Norwegian ship *Bergensfjord* docked in New York carrying two hundred cases of influenza. Four had died at sea.

In late summer, probably in Brest, France, the virus "mutated."

In the last week of August, a savagely lethal Spanish influenza exploded to life in three port cities: Brest, France; Freetown, Sierra Leone; and Boston, Massachusetts.

At the end of a calm summer, influenza returned to America—now in its most virulent form.

Chapter 2

Bewilderment

Birds, especially waterfowl, represent the Adam and Eve of influenza's genesis stories. Flu viruses develop, grow, and live—apparently harmlessly—in birds. As birds defecate on land and in water, they spread these viruses throughout the animal kingdom. Canadian lakes are a veritable witches' brew of avian influenza—each year, about 30 percent of the wild ducks preparing to migrate south from Canada carry influenza. Although influenza originates in birds, birds cannot, as far as we know, transmit flu *effectively* to human beings. A virus invades a cell by grabbing onto a "receptor," and, again, as far as we know, humans do not possess *efficient* receptors for avian flu. Other animals often serve as a "bridge species" between birds and people. Pigs, for instance. Pigs seem especially vulnerable to infection by multiple viruses at once from a myriad of species: ducks, swine, humans, chickens.

Some viruses, such as the polio virus, remain prodigiously stable over time. A polio vaccine will prove just as effective in the 1990s as in the 1950s. Influenza viruses, however, are infinitely volatile and erratic. They are also inconstant, fickle, and (one might say) promiscuous. Unlike the building blocks of the human body, the double-stranded, helix spirals of DNA (deoxyribonucleic acid), an influenza virus is composed of eight delicate strands of RNA (ribonucleic acid). The strands of RNA hang loosely together, like beads on a necklace. During replication, they can slip apart and recombine with other strands.

When duck and human viruses meet inside the lungs of a pig, for example, the RNA strands from the duck, the human, and the pig can mix and recombine, creating an entirely new RNA "necklace": a virus which is part-bird, part-pig, and part-human. Scientists call this process "viral sex." The fluky, inter-species combination of viruses, which spawns an entirely new viral "family," has probably been the cause of the cyclical seasons of plague which have periodically ravaged human populations.

A virus is a rod-shaped particle of nucleic acid, encased in protein. These proteins form sharp spikes (which allow them to adhere easily to the cells of the nose and throat), and come in two varieties: hemagglutinin (HA) and neuraminidase (NA). Influenza viruses are identified by the make-up of their proteinaceous shells, shells which are constantly changing. Most organisms possess elaborate mechanisms to prevent mutations in their genes. Influenza viruses, however, happily invite genetic "mistakes"— mistakes which provoke changes in the surface proteins. This process of constant evolutionary change is called "viral drift." It is because of viral drift that a new flu vaccine must be manufactured every year to spare human beings influenza's annual ills.

Since the 1970s, two influenza "families" have dominated Earth: the genetic offspring of the 1968 Hong Kong flu and the Russian flu of 1977. Each year dozens of genetic variations of these flu families exist naturally among the world's birds. Spreading from species to species, they move into the human population and change and change again, searching for new ways to thrive and elude human immunological response. When a completely new viral family is born (when hemagglutinin and neuraminidase combine in an entirely new way), the virus is said to have "shifted." Shift is—invariably and by definition—highly dangerous to man. Shift creates a virus never before encountered by the human immune system.

Virologists now believe that in or around 1918 the human influenza virus shifted. A new viral family was born. Then, in August 1918, the virus known as Spanish influenza mutated. Probably in Brest, France, the virus suffered a genetic mutation which transformed it into a lethal "super-flu" of astounding and unprecedented savagery.

None of this was known in 1918.

In 1665, the English novelist Daniel Defoe vividly recalled the horrors of London's Black Death. In his *Journal of the Plague Year*, Defoe wrote:

> The contagion despised all medicine; death raged in every corner; and had it gone on as it did then, a few weeks more would have cleared the town of all and everything that had a soul. Men everywhere began to despair; every heart failed them for fear; people were made desperate through the anguish of their souls, and the terrors of death sat in the very faces and countenances of the people.

The Black Death killed an estimated twenty-five million Europeans and thirty-seven million in Asia. Nine out of every ten people who developed the disease died. Still, the Medieval plague was probably less lethal than the fifty-year Plague of Justinian which ravaged Byzantium during the sixth century A.D. Like the Black Death, the Byzantine plague was probably bubonic—spread by the fleas which infest rats. An estimated one hundred million people perished.

Since the beginning of recorded history, waves of infectious disease have decimated human populations. In 412 B.C., the Greek physician Hippocrates described a respiratory illness which razed an entire Athenian army. The illness "broke out about Solstice" (December 22), and was preceded by windy atmospheric flux. Patients experienced frequent relapses which were "further complicated by pneumonia affections." Centuries passed. Similar maladies were mentioned in the annals of history. In 1510, attentive observers noted the cyclical and seasonal recurrence of these plagues. Epidemics struck every ten to thirty years, usually between the months of September and March. Why? In 1580, the Italian historians Domenico and Pietro Buoninsegni, believing the disease was caused by cold, or the baneful influence of the stars, gave the illness a name which stuck: influenza, which in Italian means simply "influence." Doctors had little to offer victims of influenza. Patients were treated with lime juice, tobacco juice, emetics (to induce vomiting), purgatives (to evacuate the bowels), or the ever-popular venesection: bled until they were pale, limp, and anemic. In 1647, influenza arrived in North America from Valencia, Spain. In the eighteenth century, American lexicographer Noah Webster lamented this "epidemic and pestilential disease." He mused that "The causes most probably exist in the elements, fire, air, and water. It is evidently the effect of some insensible qualities of the atmosphere . . . an electrical quality."

In the nineteenth century, the pace of scientific discovery quickened. Knowledge of the human body expanded greatly, largely because of the improved lenses of microscopes. In 1839, the German physiologist Theodor Schwann established that tissues were composed of cells; in 1858, Rudolf Virchow published his seminal work, *Cellular Pathology*. But what caused disease? "Miasmata," many scientists believed—"tiny living creatures" which inhabited the human body and reacted with "atmospheric poisons." With the germ theory of disease (the idea that germs cause disease), the French chemist Louis Pasteur dispelled the hypothesis of miasmata and effectively established the science of bacteriology. His discovery that the multiplication of bacteria and other microorganisms caused the fermentation of milk and wine led to the critically-important process of pasteurization, which rids milk, other dairy products, wine, and beer of disease-producing bacteria. In 1879, the celebrated German microbiologist Robert Koch proved that bacteria were the cause, not the consequence, of disease. He established the bacterial origins of anthrax, typhoid, tuberculosis, and cholera. Over the next two decades, the microbial culprits for at least twenty-one serious diseases were identified, diseases which included pneumonia, tetanus, meningitis, and gonorrhea. In 1902, Charles Richet and Pierre Portier established the concept of immunization. By the inducing of a mild, harmless episode of disease (with a vaccine), a person becomes immune to that disease. Vaccines soon became the "magic bullets" of microbiology.

The field of medicine was in ascension. Still, influenza's pernicious cycles continued in 1857, 1874, and 1890. The men of medicine watched, mystified, daunted, and enthralled. Some blamed the massive ash-plumes of Mount Krakatoa's 1883 eruption. Others echoed suspicions from centuries past—that the key to these plagues lay in the heavens, in "cosmic dust." Despite the rich advances in scientific discovery, medicine was still, by today's standards, a very young science. There was no penicillin, no antibiotic treatment for most common bacterial infections. Discovery of the bacteria responsible for tuberculosis had not led to a cure. "Sanitarians" preached the gospel of hygiene and cleanliness, but their crusade only mystified most of the world's population. Germs, if one even believed in them, were an inevitable hazard of poverty. Most tenements in America's crowded cities lacked plumbing; sewage was simply hurled into alleys. Restauranteurs used scraps off customers' plates in soup stock, then stored these fecund brews in lukewarm iceboxes. Children slept three or four to a bed. Tuberculosis, yellow fever, and polio thrived. Writer Jack Fincher's uncle died of Spanish influenza in October 1918.

> My uncle's death was but one small, sad design in the vast tap-estry of a fatally infectious disease as common to the fabric of American family life then as it is rare today. Times were so dif-ferent then. Grown-ups and children were so quickly sub-tracted from the world by so many diseases that we no longer have to fear. My grandmother, for instance, died before Wright [Fincher's uncle]. She sewed her tubercular sister's burial shroud and then died of the disease herself. Her youngest son was born tubercular. He died before his mother.

Still, the dawn of the twentieth century was a period of great optimism in medical science. Each year brought new discoveries about the cause and treatment of disease. Vaccines for smallpox, anthrax, rabies, tetanus, diphtheria; the identification of Pfeiffer's bacillus; and the control, through improved sanitation, of diseases like yellow fever, cholera, and malaria impressed the general pub-lic as well as the white-coated priests of medicine. Recent medical triumphs had given scientists a sense of invincibility.

What could be glimpsed through the lens of a microscope was no longer a secret. What was no longer a secret, what science could see, science could decipher. A handful of medical re-searchers suspected the existence of even more minuscule, invisible microorganisms, so called "filterable agents," but micro-biologists were preoccupied with bacteria. And why investigate Pfeiffer's bacillus any further?

Influenza ranked a lowly tenth among the world's leading causes of disease.

In America, Boston was where the dying started. On August 27,

1918, three sailors fell sick with Spanish influenza at Boston's Commonwealth Pier, a crowded Navy barracks housing some seven thousand men. The next day, 8 new cases appeared. The next, 58. The disease was stunningly contagious. On day four of the outbreak, 81 fell ill; on day five, 106. Patients transferred to Chelsea Naval Hospital infected the physicians who admitted them. Physical collapse was shockingly swift. Men went from robust health to complete prostration in a matter of hours. Fevers soared to 105 degrees. Five to 10 percent of patients developed secondary pneumonia which in 70 percent of cases proved fatal. Soon, two thousand men of the First Naval District were desperately sick with influenza. On September 3, the first civilian casualty of Spanish influenza was admitted to Boston City Hospital. Still, no one of importance seemed to notice that a stunningly infectious disease was on the loose. That same day, four thousand men marched through Boston in a "Win-the-War-for-Freedom" parade. Eight days later, before a wild throng at Fenway Park, Babe Ruth led the Boston Red Sox to victory in the World Series. That same day, three men dropped dead on the sidewalks of nearby Quincy.

On September 13, the *Boston Globe* declared that doctors had the Spanish flu "pretty well in hand." That afternoon, the Navy announced 163 new cases. "No reason to be alarmed," a Rear Admiral declared.

A chill rain started falling on New England. In military bases all around Boston, soldiers continued to get sick. Camp Devens, a sprawling army base just west of Boston, suffered 12,604 cases of flu in just two weeks. The Camp hospital, built to accommodate two thousand patients, was grappling with eight thousand. Some victims collapsed outside in the rain, waiting to be admitted. In ward after ward, ashen-faced soldiers lay on bloody sheets, delirious and dying. Overwhelmed nurses triaged patients by looking at their feet. A man with black feet was considered as good as dead. The statistics were staggering: 29.6 percent of the

Thirteenth Battalion was sick, 17.3 percent of the Forty-second Infantry, and 24.6 percent of the Trains and Military Police. Every day, dozens of men died.

In mid September, the Surgeon General wired for help from Colonel Victor Vaughan, a distinguished epidemiologist, and Dr. William Henry Welch, the renowned dean of American medicine. At sixty-eight, Welch was a handsome, impressive man with a white mustache and goatee. America's preeminent physician as well as its most influential scientist, Welch was the living embodiment of the rising power of medical science.

But Camp Devens, like a scene out of fourteenth-century Europe, gave the great men a shock. Later, Vaughan would describe "a picture painted on my memory cells":

> I see hundreds of young, stalwart men in uniform coming into the wards of the hospital...every bed is full, yet others crowd in. The faces wear a bluish cast; a cough brings up the blood-stained sputum. In the morning the dead bodies are stacked about the morgue like cord wood.

Even Welch, veteran of decades of gruesome pathologic analysis, "was excited and nervous." When an autopsy revealed sodden, blue, swollen lungs, Dr. Welch turned and said, "This must be some new kind of infection." Then Welch chose a terrifying word. "Or plague," he added. A murmur ran through the room.

Dr. Rufus Cole, who had accompanied Welch, later recalled, "It was the only time I ever saw Dr. Welch really worried and disturbed." Neither Vaughan nor Welch had anything to offer the dying soldiers at Camp Devens. On September 23, the day of their visit, sixty-three men died. Within weeks, Camp Devens would count seventeen thousand ill; 768 soldiers died.

Still, to most Bostonians, the epidemic remained strangely remote. Children like Francis Russell in Miss Sykes' third grade class hardly noticed. It was a disease for soldiers and sailors only, wasn't it? Francis Russell later wrote:

> To our confident immortality, influenza seemed no threat at all, rather one more incident in the excitement of the war's climax. At recess time, girls jumped rope and sang:
> I had a little bird
> And its name was Enza
> I opened the window and
> In-flew-enza.

The lungs are truly airy organs: the lightest organs in the human body. Wispy as a butterfly's wing, buoyant as a soap bubble, they seem hardly up to their task—a lifetime of stubborn, unceasing breaths. With each inhale and exhale, each breathy excursion, the lungs' 750 million tiny air sacs (alveoli) exchange the blood's gaseous wastes for fresh oxygen. Any injury to their delicate tissue impedes this critical renewal. With pneumonia, the elastic tissue of the lungs becomes coarse, riddled with hard nodules, but this takes time, or it usually does. Not so with Spanish influenza. Autopsies of patients who died within forty-eight hours after onset of the disease revealed heavy, swollen, bloody lungs which, incredibly, sank in water. The lungs were literally bleeding. A thin, frothy liquid oozed up the throat. As rigor mortis set in, blood gushed from the nose.

What was causing this catastrophic failure? What *was* Spanish influenza? Some medical men guessed pneumonic plague, like the medieval Black Death. Between 1910 and 1917, pneumonic plague had killed scores of people in Manchuria and China. Perhaps Chinese laborers, seeking work in America and France, had brought this plague with them. Or perhaps Spanish influenza was the child of war. Europe's "Sausage Machine" had created unprecedented carnage and technological violence: mustard gas, thousands of tons of explosives, corpses left to rot in the open air. Perhaps Europe's polluted atmosphere was revisiting its poisons upon the human race.

Like a runaway train, the epidemic was gathering steam. "The whole city is stricken," a Gloucester nurse wrote. "We were taken quite unawares." From Boston, the flu pushed westward, just as the pioneers had; in fact, it followed the pioneer trails, which were now railroads. From the Northeastern seaboard, it traveled to the cities of the Midwest, then the Far West. Crowded army camps, with traffic back and forth from flu-ridden Europe, became home bases for the plague.

Doctors often could not diagnose the mysterious disease, let alone cure it. The first cases at Camp Devens were treated as cerebrospinal meningitis; the illness was simply too explosive, and too violent for "flu." From all over the world—Australia, Russia, India, South America—reports were coming in of weird, sinister complications. Influenza patients were developing cataracts, vertigo, enlarged spleens, gangrene of the sexual organs. Purple blisters appeared on blue, oxygen-starved skin. Some autopsies revealed the cause of death as asphyxia of the alveoli: bloody lungs had literally suffocated from lack of oxygen. There were other findings, too, pathologic findings never before associated with influenza: leucopenia—where the blood becomes deficient in white cells; deafness; blindness; and coma. Baltimore's Dr. John F. Hogan recorded: "[A]nother type of case became totally unconscious hours or even days before the end, restless in his coma, with head thrown back, mouth half open, a ghastly pallor of the cyanosed face, purple lips and ears—a dreadful sight."

As the epidemic spread, influenza was variously diagnosed as chlorine gas poisoning, Asiatic cholera, scarlet fever, typhoid, food poisoning, and appendicitis. Doctors simply did not know what to think. Was this horrific disease really just the flu? The strange disease even felt mysterious. The first "symptom," often, was a sudden sense of awe—a fear people could not explain, even to themselves.

It was mysterious and it was quick. "In the midst of perfect health," one doctor wrote, "the patient would be seized rapidly, almost suddenly, with a sense of such prostration as to be utterly unable to carry on." In Rio de Janeiro, one man asked another where the streetcar stopped, thanked him politely, then fell over dead. On a Cape Town trolley, the driver, conductor, and five passengers collapsed and died within a three-mile stretch of road. In London's overwhelmed Middlesex Hospital, Dr. Robert Parry could only "direct traffic," sending the sick to the emergency ward or the morgue. A San Francisco secretary, Henrietta Burt, spent an evening playing bridge. "We played long after midnight. When we left, we were all apparently well. By 8 o'clock in the morning, I was too ill to get out of bed, and the friend at whose house we played was dead." The physician and poet, William Carlos Williams, recorded, "They'd be sick one day and gone the next, just like that, fill up and die."

In the New England town of Brockton, Massachusetts, eight thousand people—20 percent of the city's population—fell sick. Mayor William L. Gleason mobilized the town, even using the Boy Scouts as messengers and errand-boys. Still, the contagion spread. Dr. Carl Holmberg, chairman of Brockton's beleaguered Board of Health, told a nurse that battling Spanish influenza was like "fighting with a ghost."

One morning, a young woman, seven months pregnant, arrived at Brockton Hospital. Bloody fluid was already accumulating in her lungs. A nurse remembered:

> The baby was born prematurely and died at birth, but I did not dare tell the mother it had died. She kept begging me to see her baby. . . . I assured her that he was fine and beautiful and she would hold him as soon as she was stronger. She had such a lovely look on her face as she talked about her son, and how happy her husband would be. It was an effort for her to talk as her lungs were filling. . . . She died late that after-

noon. I put the baby into her arms and fixed them so that they seemed only to be sleeping. And so the husband saw them when he came.

The friendly, perfumed street in Philadelphia where Anna Milani lived was changing. Anna and her brothers and sisters still marched down Ninth Street to St. Nicholas Church, trombone blaring, singing: "I Spy Kaiser at the Door. We'll get a lemon pie, and we'll squash him in his eye, and there won't be any Kaiser anymore." But lemon pie no longer seemed weapon enough against Kaiser Bill. Philadelphia's sons were returning from Europe in coffins. Anna Milani recalls:

We thought our boys would go over there and fight the Germans and then come home heroes. But boys were coming home in coffins. So many boys on our street died. In one house, the boy who'd been killed was an only child. His father was so filled with grief he shot himself. His wife began screaming and we all started running towards the house. People were shouting: "Mr. Merino killed himself because he couldn't stand the thought of his son dying. He couldn't stand to see his son in a casket draped with the American flag."

And something other than war was affecting Anna Milani's neighborhood. The mysterious plague was moving closer. People were swiftly, strangely, tragically dying. Across the street, a teenage girl died.

I remember it was a mild day and we were sitting outside on the steps. Around twilight, we heard screams. In that same house, the same family where the girl had died, an eighteen-month-old baby died. Someone told us there was an epidemic of Spanish influenza: *Influenza de la Spagnuolo*.

In North Carolina, seven-year-old Dan Tonkel's simple, peaceful life was changing. His schemes to earn nickels for his beloved ice cream and his apprenticeship with Miss Leah in the yard goods department of his father's clothing store were a thing of the past. This simple community, without radios, televisions, or parks, was suddenly, inexplicably changing. No more Saturday morning farmers' market. No more weekly movie at Goldsboro's theater. Schools closed.

> Now, that's a big event in the life of an elementary school child. We were thrilled about schools closing, but a few days later, my father said, "Son, I want you to go to work with me." I asked him why and he said there was a flu going around and all his employees were home sick or in the hospital. From then on, I went to work with him. We had to shut down the whole second floor of the store—ladies ready-to-wear and our big millinery department—which was a momentous decision. Business was very, very sparse.
>
> Then my father told me already three of his eight employees had died. He told me, "Miss Leah will not be coming back." I said, "Why not?" He said, "Because Leah died." Miss Leah was the first of his employees to die.
>
> I was old enough to understand what death was. I suddenly realized what was happening, that many of our good friends and people who loved us were going to die.

Most tragedies have their Cassandra: the prophet whose warnings are disbelieved. This story is no exception.

Rupert Blue was America's chief public health officer, Surgeon General of the United States. A husky, genial native of North Carolina, Blue had worn the royal-blue threads of the Public Health Service for twenty-six years. He had beaten bubonic plague in San Francisco and yellow fever in New Orleans, and had thrived among the microbes and the shadowy commerce of the steamy French Quarter and San Francisco's Barbary Coast. When William Gorgas sailed for France, Blue assumed command of America's 180 Health Officers and 44 quarantine stations. An affable, down-home sort, he filled his Washington office with the nation's medical elite as well as the ragged rat-catchers and ditch diggers from his colorful past.

On September 17, 1918, Blue shot a terse telegram to the Health Officers of the nation's forty-eight states: "Request all information regarding the prevalence of influenza in your State." The scope of this epidemic already dwarfed anything Blue had ever seen. New England was completely engulfed in flu; across the country, hundreds of people were dying. On September 13, the official number of afflicted soldiers (by conservative estimate) rose above twenty thousand. Obviously, the virus was traveling the routes of the infected military and sparking outbreaks among the civilian population. Containment was crucial. Blue suggested the Armed Forces immediately halt shipment of sick soldiers or those exposed to the virus and quickly remove healthy troops from infected zones. But Blue, Surgeon General of the world's most powerful nation, had little actual authority. He could only advise, warn, cajole, and entreat. He could not force cooperation; he could only ask for it. Movement of troops continued.

Across the nation, physicians and citizens alike were flummoxed. Correct diagnosis of this bewildering disease was critical. But what *was* it? Blue released a bulletin to the press. The plainspoken simplicity of Blue's communiqué could not disguise his own puzzlement:

> In appearance one is struck by the fact that the patient looks sick. Ordinarily the fever lasts from three to four days and the

patient recovers. When death occurs, it is usually the result of the development of a pneumonia or of some other complication.

For the sick, Blue recommended bed rest, good food, aspirin, salts of quinine. He suggested the widespread adoption of surgical masks—gauzy masks which covered the mouth and nose—by people nursing the sick. Soon laymen and officials across the nation decided that what was sensible in the sickroom was just as sensible everywhere. Sale of face masks exploded. Sewn by America's women or manufactured by Levi-Strauss, featured in department stores or distributed by the Red Cross, masks became a ubiquitous sight on America's streets, worn by policemen, socialites, barbers, and newlyweds. On October 4, Blue sent another missive to the Health Officers of the nation's states. He asked authorities to "close all public gathering places if the community is threatened with the epidemic. This will do much towards checking the spread of the disease."

Like other members of the medical elite, Blue had little else to offer. The Public Health Service possessed only a handful of doctors and researchers and was wholly unprepared for a disaster of such magnitude. Blue asked the Health Officers of each state to mobilize local efforts and report to him daily about the progress of the disease. But state health officials were overwhelmed and information on the spread of the epidemic through the civilian population remained sketchy. Today, the Public Health Service's annual budget tops thirteen billion dollars. Its staff, including Civil Service doctors, technicians, and scientists, numbers upwards of forty-seven thousand. Because of such powerful entities as the Centers for Disease Control in Atlanta and the National Institute of Allergy and Infectious Disease, its pervasive scrutiny is felt in local clinics throughout the nation and the world. Blue, by comparison, had an annual budget of less than three million dollars, a sum considered meager even at the time. As Boston wired asking for five hundred physicians and other stricken localities made similar requests, Blue came up against the implacable reality of the war. Some 50,000 of America's 140,000 physicians were in Europe. Nurses were in even shorter supply.

On September 12, the American Expeditionary Force commenced its first major offensive. The A.E.F. blasted through the German lines at St. Mihiel, outside Verdun, France. In truth, the Germans were in the process of withdrawing troops from St. Mihiel in order to strengthen their forces elsewhere. Nevertheless, in two days, fifteen thousand German soldiers and 250 guns were captured and seven thousand Germans were killed in what seemed a dramatic American victory. British Prime Minister David Lloyd George, sick with Spanish influenza, dispatched a congratulatory cable to Pershing: "The news came to me on my sick bed: it was better and infinitely more palatable than any physic." Victory was within reach if the Allied pressure continued. On September 26, the Allies' most massive offensive began. The A.E.F and supporting French divisions scrambled from their trenches into a swirling fog of dust and gassy smoke, and began smashing into German lines in the Meuse-Argonne sector. It was a massive effort. The U.S. Army expended more ammunition in the battle of Meuse-Argonne than was used by the Union Army in the entire Civil War. Although the Allies were immediately stalled and the Front transformed into a gassy, bomb-cratered wasteland of human and military debris, American newspapers went wild; the public could think of little else. Still, six thousand miles from the bloody battlefields of France, in the peaceful state of Massachusetts, some fifty thousand citizens were morbidly sick with influenza. On September 26, the day the Meuse-Argonne offensive began, 156 Bostonians died of influenza. Massachusetts' chief Health Officer wired Surgeon General Blue for help. Massachusetts Governor Calvin Coolidge sent pleas to President Woodrow Wilson, the Mayor of Toronto, and the governors of Vermont, Maine, and Rhode Island. He reported, "Our doctors and nurses are being thoroughly mobilized and worked to the limit. . . . Many cases receive no attention whatever."

On September 19, Massachusetts organized a State Emergency Health Committee. Liberty Loan parades were postponed. The Stock Exchange slashed its hours in half. Theaters closed. Athletic events were canceled. Sunday, September 22 was proclaimed a churchless Sunday. In Quincy's shipyard, the staccato noise of riveters died out into a cacophony of coughs, then near silence. Should schools close or remain open? In slum areas, schools were often less crowded and, therefore, safer for children than home. Schools, however, were needed as emergency hospitals and soup kitchens. Local officials were left to decide.

In the Dorchester section of Boston, the stucco schoolhouse where Francis Russell was attending third grade remained open. The school lay on the route to New Cavalry cemetery. By now, funeral processions had become nearly continuous.

Coffins were piling up in the yard of the cemetery. John "Pigeye" Mulvey, who owned the land, pitched a circus tent next to the funeral chapel to hide the coffins. Francis Russell later mused: "The tent lay there white and billowing, like some grotesque autumn carnival among the withered leaves, with the somber line of vehicles trailing through New Calvary gate." The cemetery was literally becoming undone. Caskets buried in shallow graves, one on top of the other, were rising out of the muddy ground.

All day long, in Miss Sykes' classroom, Francis Russell watched and listened.

As we followed the morning routine of multiplication tables, we could hear the carriages passing outside, the clop of horses' hooves in the wet leaves.... The plague stretched out its fingertips toward Miss Sykes. Trying as best she could to conceal it from us, she became sharp and tense-voiced. The rattle of the hacks had broken her nerve. In the afternoon the sun's rays would strike against the glass of a passing carriage and reflect waveringly across the ceiling of our room, and we, distracted by light and sound, would crane toward the row of windows. "Eyes front!" she would shriek at us. For the fear was on her.

Chapter 3

Rumors, Confusion, Denial

Hope springs eternal in the human heart, and no one is more hopeful than an ambitious politician. On August 12, 1918, when the flu-ridden Norwegian ship *Bergensfjord* docked in New York, Health Commissioner Dr. Royal Copeland reacted to the news of the ship's contagion with an optimism which was both resolute and misguided. "The city is in no danger of an epidemic," Copeland announced. Rumors of four passengers buried at sea and two hundred removed to Brooklyn hospitals (Mrs. Jensine Olsen, the fifth victim, died immediately upon arrival) spread quickly through the boroughs. Copeland reassured the public: the passengers from the ill-fated *Bergensfjord* were suffering from pneumonia, not Spanish influenza. No need for quarantine or even an isolation ward. Copeland was a implacable optimist and he was not about to take a household disease seriously. An eye specialist, untrained in Public Health, Copeland had only recently become Health Commissioner of New York. He had swelling political ambitions; eventually, he became a U.S. Senator. Influenza, Copeland suggested, resulted mostly from malnutrition and the poor hygiene of Europeans. "You haven't heard of our doughboys getting it, have you? You bet you haven't, and you won't. No need for our people to worry over the matter."

Royal Copeland was not the only public official to react to

news of the burgeoning epidemic with cheerful denial and a
brash, steadfast belief in his locality's immunity. Most health officials considered the puzzling outbreak Boston's problem. A Baltimore commissioner said, "There is no special reason to fear an
outbreak of disease in our city." What was happening in New
England seemed strangely unreal. Reports of influenza—the *flu*
turned deadly, into a lethal, medieval-like plague—must be ex-
aggerated. How could "plague" strike us now? How could
"plague" exist in modern times, the age of the radio crystal oscil-
lator and the high-speed hydrofoil? After all, the "epidemic" was
only a few soldiers getting sick. Like medical men and the general public, American politicians were incredulous. Perhaps if
they disbelieved it, the danger would simply go away. Perhaps if
they did nothing, the danger would vanish. The war, of course,
was more important.

As flu enveloped the nation, so did denial, false hopes, rumors,
confusion, and paranoia. Chicago officials declared, "We have
the Spanish influenza situation well in hand." The head of San
Francisco's Board of Health announced that he doubted the flu
would reach his city at all. Like officials in Philadelphia, Seattle,
Santa Fe, and New Orleans, he claimed his city's "ideal climate"
would keep the flu away. "If ordinary precautions are observed,
there is no cause for alarm," said the chief health officer of Los
Angeles. Two days later, influenza forced the closure of all L.A.'s
schools, theaters, and churches. Partly to avoid panic, partly because the war was all-consuming, newspapers remained fixed on
news from France. American cartoonists portrayed the deadly illness as a quaintly-wizened figure, "Old Man Grippe." A doctor in
Arizona revealed a typical blindness towards his own statistics.
He reported "[f]ifty cases of influenza, all mild. Four deaths."

For many of the same reasons, the response of the Federal government mirrored those of locals officials. The recommendations

of Surgeon Generals William Gorgas and Rupert Blue and the grave concerns of Doctors Vaughan and Welch and others remained largely untranslated into action. It was difficult to mobilize against something so inscrutable, so unbelievable, so difficult to pinpoint. The United States was already facing a very real and visible enemy: Erich von Ludendorff's divisions in the forests of the Argonne. The European War was insistent, terrifying, and exhilarating. It was the nation's, and Woodrow Wilson's, pervasive and overwhelming priority. America's military machine was driven not just by the demands of General Pershing and French Marshal Foch, but by the weight of its own massive momentum, a momentum which propelled it hurtling forward throughout September, even as influenza engulfed the Armed Forces. Recruits were rushed into crowded army camps, where they promptly got sick. Clearly, Spanish influenza thrived among the cramped ranks of the military. Just as clearly, the public was becoming infected where the military and public intersected. But Rupert Blue's alerts to public health officials, his bulletins to the Press, and his appeals to the military brass for quarantine and judicious movement of troops fell largely on the deaf ears of people too preoccupied, incredulous, or blithely disbelieving to hear. Troop trains crisscrossing America remained hideously overcrowded. Three men were crammed into every double seat. In sleeper cars, two soldiers often shared one small berth. On September 26, the 328th Labor Battalion left Louisiana with 12 men sick with influenza. Three days later, when the Battalion arrived in Newport News, Virginia, 120 men were sick. Soon, 61 more succumbed. The crowded train ride cost the 328th Labor Battalion 181 men. The seas were equally perilous. Corpse after corpse was lowered over the side of heaving vessels, draped in the American flag. A sailor on the *Wilhemina* watched the plank tip, and flag-wrapped bodies drop into the ocean. "I confess I was near to tears, and there was a tightening around my throat," he wrote. "It was death, death in one of its worst forms, to be consigned nameless to the sea."

In *Epidemic and Peace, 1918*, the pandemic's distinguished historian, Alfred Crosby, writes:

> The people of the United States were stark raving patriotic in summer 1918. The interweaving of the war and the pandemic makes what from a distance of a half-century seems to be a pattern of complete insanity. On September 11, Washington officials disclosed to reporters their fear that Spanish influenza had arrived, and on the next day thirteen million men of precisely the ages most liable to die of Spanish influenza and its complications lined up all over the United States and crammed into city halls, post offices, and school houses to register for the draft. It was a gala flag-waving affair everywhere, including Boston, where ninety-six thousand registered and sneezed and coughed on one another.

Blindness prevailed all over the country. In late September, mammoth bond and Liberty Loan drives drew hundreds of thousands, sick and well, into America's streets. Hoards gathered in rainy Chicago. 150,000 sardined into the streets of San Francisco. Hundreds of thousands marched in Philadelphia.

In the autumn of 1918, Philadelphia was a crammed, expanding city, with swelling ghettos of newly-arrived immigrants and Southern blacks, a Naval Yard, and two nearby Army camps: Camp Dix in New Jersey and Camp Meade in Maryland. On September 11, influenza appeared in Philadelphia's Naval Shipyard and days later, in Camp Dix and Camp Meade. Despite the example of devastated Boston, Dr. Wilmer Krusen of Philadelphia's Department of Health and Charities and Dr. A. A. Cairns of the Bureau of Health assured the public it was unlikely that the disease would reach the city's civilian population. Navy officials announced they were working "to confine this disease to its present limits, and in this we are sure to be successful." On September 21, Dr. Paul A. Lewis of the Phipps Institute of Philadelphia announced he had isolated the source of the flu: Pfeiffer's bacillus. All seemed well. According to the *Philadelphia Inquirer*, Dr. Lewis' discovery had "armed the medical profession with absolute knowledge on which to base its campaign against this disease." So on September 28, two hundred thousand people marched through Philadelphia in the Fourth Liberty Loan Drive parade.

The parade stretched for twenty-three blocks. It was a beautiful autumn day. People linked arms and sang patriotic songs. Planes flew overhead; antiaircraft guns fired "at" the marchers. Women in mourning were drawn from the crowd and held up as examples: "This woman gave her all. What will you give?" During each pause, the crowd was entreated, pressured, and harangued to buy bonds. Why buy bonds? Why send "our darlings" to France? "You have brought them into the soul-awakening experience of War for Principle. They must be *kept* there, equipped for this stupendous task, until the task is finished. *And your support is the only thing that will do it.*"

Even children got into the act. Susanna Turner and Columba Voltz were two faces in Philadelphia's patriotic crowd. Susanna Turner was seventeen years old, a student at William Penn High School. "We were so conscious of the war, of liberty. We marched and sang, and saved our money for Liberty Bonds." Columba Voltz was eight, the daughter of a tailor. To Columba, the Liberty Loan parade was "a marvelous singing fest, with huge posters of Uncle Sam bobbing through the crowd." Columba linked arms with her friend, Katherine, singing, "Over There, Over There" and "I Never Raised my Son to be a Soldier." She and Katherine had saved their pennies. Twenty-five pennies bought a Thrift Stamp; a five dollar book of Thrift Stamps bought a War Bond. "Katherine and I were happy, thinking we were helping the war effort." In his tailor's shop near Rittenhouse Square, Columba's father was helping the war effort, too.

> My father sewed costumes for masquerade balls which were held at the Bellevue Stratford Hotel to raise money for the war. I remember peering through the railing, watching him measure people for their costumes. One costume which was especially magnificent was of a wooden soldier. When the man came for his final fitting and put on the costume, he looked just like a wooden soldier. He marched back and forth across the room.

No one wanted to curtail the war effort or shut down the huge, perilous displays of patriotism. No one wanted to suggest life should change. No one wanted to believe that the flu could actually come to their town. Partly to avoid panic, partly because the war was so electrifying, most newspapers remained dominated by news of Europe. But small ads were beginning to appear in the nation's newspapers: "Spanish influenza! Can you afford sudden death? If not, protect your Family by Life Insurance."

Like most people, a striking, black-haired reporter in Denver named Katherine Anne Porter was not much concerned with someone else being sick. She had other things on her mind. Porter would become a well-known writer; her novel *Ship of Fools* and her short story "Pale Horse, Pale Rider" are considered American classics. In 1918, Porter was a young newspaper woman in love with an army lieutenant. A largely autobiographical story, "Pale Horse, Pale Rider" captures the mood of that eerie Indian summer. "Miranda" (Porter herself) awakened hearing the word: "War." All day long, the word echoed in her mind, "reminding her of what she forgot happily in sleep, and only in sleep." Every day, self-styled "patriots" visited the newspaper office, badgering her to buy Liberty Bonds. That Miranda earned only eighteen dollars a week was, the patriots insisted, "no excuse, no excuse at all, and you know it, with the Huns overrunning martyred Belgium...with our American boys fighting and dying in Belleau Wood." But Miranda wanted to forget the war. She wanted simply to be in love with her lieutenant, Adam. And to Miranda, like most Americans, the deadly epidemic still seemed remote. She and Adam strolled through town...

> They paused at another corner, under a half-foliaged maple, and hardly glanced at a funeral procession approaching... Adam said, "The men are dying like flies out there, anyway. This funny new disease. Simply knocks you into a cocked hat."
> "Seems to be a plague," said Miranda, "something out of the Middle Ages. Did you ever see so many funerals, ever?"

America was not alone in her tunnel vision. In 1918, in no nation on Earth was influenza a reportable disease. Many countries lacked even a central Department of Health. The influenza epidemic of 1889–90 had killed thousands of Britons. Nevertheless, in 1918, influenza was not one of Britain's nineteen "notifiable" diseases. As in America, the early warnings of Britain's medical experts were lost amid the drama and exigencies of war. On August 10, Britain's Medical Research Council, tracking influenza's "spring wave" through Europe, had predicted a second, deadlier epidemic in the fall. The Council's urgent call for research and collaboration among bacteriologists went largely unheard. A top British officer told the Council's Secretary, Walter Fletcher: "Damn research, sir—we've got to get on with the war." Another who failed to heed the Council's warnings was Britain's highest public health official, Chief Medical Officer Sir Arthur Newsholme. Alerted to the danger, Newsholme shot a memo to local authorities, ordering them to prevent crowding on trams and buses, asking factories to stagger work hours. Then, fearing panic and a drop-off in arms production, Newsholme changed his mind. He withdrew his recommendations.

Eventually, 228,000 Britons died of Spanish influenza.

> There didn't seem to be any reason to think of the plague ever having to do with us. But in a gradual, remorseless way, it kept moving closer and closer. I know my parents were worried. I paid less attention to their words than to the sound of their voices. When they discussed it, I heard anxiety.
>
> —William Maxwell of Lincoln, Illinois

> We heard stories, lots of stories. We heard about what was happening in Boston, but people didn't want to believe they could be healthy in the morning and dead by nightfall. There were lots of rumors, especially that Germans had planted the germs of the disease.
>
> —Bill Sardo of Washington, D.C.

In 1918, American brewers of beer and ale placed an eye-catching ad in the *Boston Evening Transcript* and a half-dozen other papers across the country. The ad read: "In the many acts of disloyalty discovered by the Department of Justice prior to and during the war, there is not one single instance where any brewer, directly or indirectly, has in any way been found guilty of any act which could be considered disloyal." Patriotic Americans were a suspicious lot, and the Germanic names and origins of beer and ale brought even the nation's most cherished beverages under suspicion of treason. The Spanish Lady (already, by her very name, casting aspersions on unlucky Spaniards) was not immune from anti-German sentiment and paranoia.

On September 18, Lieutenant Colonel Philip S. Doane, chief of the Health and Sanitation Section of the Emergency Fleet

Corporation, suggested America had become infected with germs spread by Germans "put ashore from U-boats." Doane's suspicions appeared in newspapers across the nation:

> It would be quite easy for one of these German agents to turn loose Spanish influenza germs in a theater or some other place where large numbers of persons are assembled. The Germans have started epidemics in Europe, and there is no reason why they should be particularly gentle with America.

Anxious Americans agreed. A woman in Socorro, New Mexico, insisted that German sympathizers had poisoned the local drinking water. A man in Passaic, New Jersey, believed Huns had planted germs in cigarettes. In "Pale Horse, Pale Rider," a reporter wryly passes on the rumors:

> "They say," said Towney, "that it is really caused by germs brought by a German ship to Boston, a camouflaged ship . . . the germs were sprayed over the city. . . . Somebody reported seeing a strange, thick, greasy-looking cloud float up out of Boston Harbor and spread slowly all over that end of town."

Rumors of a German plot failed to account for the fact that "*Blitzkatarrh*" had crippled the German army in the spring. Autumn's even more lethal strain was continuing to do so; this microbial "secret weapon" eventually killed more than 225,000 Germans. Still, fearful Americans were eager to find someone besides the noncombatant Spanish to blame for this mysterious plague. But did the plague even exist? Perhaps it was a figment of our collective imagination. One Missouri official dismissed reports of the epidemic as "Hun propaganda." To the flamboyant evangelist (and ex-White Sox ballplayer) Billy Sunday, Spanish influenza was a "German ploy." "The whole thing is part of their propaganda; it started over there in Spain, where they scattered germs around.... There's nothing short of hell they haven't stooped to do since the war began. Darn their hides!"

For Sunday and others, the Germans were behind the outbreak. For others, it was caused by something as old and simple as sin. The *New York Post* declared: "Epidemics are the punishment which nature inflicts for the violation of her laws." Jehovah's witnesses considered the epidemic the realization of Jesus' prophesy on the Mount of Olives, the predicted time of "pestilence and sorrows." If sin was the lightning rod for influenza's strike, would not good Christian people be spared? The people in Harriet Ferrel's Philadelphia neighborhood thought so. When Pentecostal preachers sermonized on the corner of Fairmont and Brooklyn Streets, predicting an imminent calamity, Harriet's neighbors had ignored them. Cleanliness was next to Godliness. Like tuberculosis, which ravaged the poor, Spanish influenza was probably a "lower class disease." Even New York's Health Commissioner, Dr. Royal Copeland, had wrongly linked influenza with malnutrition and the "poor hygiene of Europeans."

Evangelist Billy Sunday changed his message from "Hun espionage" to sin. He preached to a huge crowd in Providence, Rhode Island. Sin was the cause, and prayer the answer. "We can meet here tonight and pray down the epidemic," Sunday said. But even as he spoke, members of his audience collapsed with flu and were carried from the hall. New York's Christian Scientists offered yet another interpretation. They called the relative health of the city's Chinese population the result of "mind over matter." What the Chinese could not read about in English-speaking newspapers, they would not catch.

For millions of inner-city poor, the scourge of influenza was compounded by a myriad of other hazards. In 1911, a noted commentator on things American, British ambassador Lord James Bryce, had declared, "The government of the cities is the one conspicuous failure of the United States." Social Progressives had targeted the nation's teeming slums, but to minimal effect. As influenza engulfed America's cities, its spread was kindled not only by overcrowding and poor hygiene, but also by confusion. Language barriers, ethnic differences, and the conflicting agendas of immigrant and native created distrust, puzzlement, and, not infrequently, chaotic misunderstanding. To many European and Asian immigrants, the baneful effects of poor hygiene and overcrowding—the gospel according to white, English-speaking officials—was difficult to comprehend and, in the face of extreme poverty, an ultimately pointless notion. Efforts were made. Cities published circulars in a score of languages. In Boston, Health Department flyers were issued in Italian and Yiddish; one Pennsylvania mining company published anti-flu bulletins in six languages. Still, breakdowns occurred. When a vessel docked in New York City, twenty-five sick Chinese sailors were removed to the Municipal Lodging House. Terrified by their white-masked, white-robed, English-speaking hosts, the Chinese refused to take off their clothes for fear of being robbed. Believing the food was poisoned, they refused to eat. All but eight died. At Camp Wheeler in Macon, Georgia, fifteen hundred black recruits arrived at the railway station, then scrambled for cover, believing the masked medical orderlies on the platform were Ku Klux Klansmen. Indeed, the epidemic in some instances strained an already tense relationship between blacks and whites. In recent years, thousands of Southern blacks had flooded the manufacturing cities of the North in search of jobs; racial tensions escalated. Race riots in East St. Louis in 1917 were some of the worst in U.S. history, and riots continued through the end of the decade. In 1918, the Spanish Lady was felt deeply among marginalized populations in America's crowded slums.

In New Haven, Connecticut, John Deleno was attending first grade. There was no room at the neighborhood school, so John and his friends were taught at a local pool hall. John lived in an enclave of Italian immigrants. He remembers:

> Life to me was just lots of Italians living together. We all knew each other, we were always visiting, passing food around. We were just one big happy family. For every little affair—baptisms, birthdays, Communion—we had a party. It was always parties, parties, parties.

In 1918, John was six. He lived down the block from an undertaker. Coffins began accumulating on the sidewalk outside the mortuary. As the stacks of coffins rose higher, John and his buddies began playing on the coffins. They climbed on them, jumped from one to another.

> We thought—boy, this is great. It's like climbing the pyramids. Then one day, I slipped and fell and broke my nose on one of the coffins. My mother was very upset. She said, didn't I realize there were people in those boxes? People who had died? I couldn't understand that. Why had all these people died?

With a basket of chicken and cake, nurse Josie Mabel Brown took the Pullman from St. Louis to her assignment at the Great Lakes Naval Training Center outside Chicago.

> Someone opened a paper in front of me. I saw "six thousand have Spanish Influenza in Great Lakes, Illinois." I said, "Oh, that's where I'm going." With my heart thumping, I asked, "What is Spanish influenza?"

The state of Virginia released a bulletin to its citizens:

Q. What is influenza?
A. Influenza is a disease which starts with a chill or chilly feel-
ings, makes a person very feverish and weak, and causes a
cough, sore throat, and much aching.
Q. What other names are there for this disease?
A. Grippe, the flu, and Spanish influenza.
Q. Is influenza a new disease?
A. No.
Q. What causes influenza?
A. A tiny living poisonous plant called the germ of influenza.
Q. Has this epidemic been altogether a curse?
A. No, if we learn from this experience the lessons that we
should learn, it will mean a blessing in disguise, for it will
cause the reduction of the sick and death rate from many
other diseases.

What *was* causing this bewildering disease? New York's Dr.
Gedide Friendman pointed an accusing finger at bed bugs. The
British Twenty-third Division, stationed near the Lombard silk-
making village of Arzignano, declared the culprits were silk-
worms. J. Blaustein of Springfield, Massachusetts, reasoned the
epidemic had "come from fish. Fish swimming in poisoned, U-
boat infested waters." A stubborn Swede, determined to prove
the pandemic was the result of a world-wide pork shortage,
killed and devoured a thirty-pound suckling pig, then declared
himself immune. The *New York Herald* published the theory of
a Bostonian, Dr. Charles E. Page. Page believed only nakedness
could repulse the flu:

Influenza is caused chiefly by excessive clothing on an animal
by nature naked. The skin is a true breathing organ; its mil-

lions of blood vessels are forever gasping for air under even the lightest of drapery, while under the ordinary garb of many folds of clothing it is practically smothered and the blood is deprived of needed oxygen.

Seattle's Dr. Louis Dechmann pronounced: "Influenza is a negative disease. I am of the opinion that it would be more accurate to name this disease *panasthenia*: a general loss of vitality." To him, Spanish influenza was a pernicious descendant of the popular Victorian affliction neurasthenia. A catch-all illness characterized by loss of energy, memory, feelings of inadequacy, and general "exhaustion of the nervous system," neurasthenia was the prevalent male version of female "hysteria." During the last half of the nineteenth century, hysteria incapacitated hundreds of thousands of Victorian women, driving them into the care of perplexed and exasperated physicians with weird tics and paralyses, incorrigible hiccups, violent swooning fits, mutism, hallucinations, or deep melancholy. Just as Dr. Rudolf Virchow was penning *Cellular Pathology*, Louis Pasteur rebuking the "miasmatic" theory of disease, and Robert Koch releasing his seminal, "The Aetiology of Traumatic Infectious Disease," male neurasthenia was being treated with venisection (blood-letting) and galvanism (electrical shock and stimulation), and remedies for female hysteria included vaginal "fumigation," sexual surgery, and beatings with wet towels. Philadelphia's famous Dr. S. Weir Mitchell, doctor to presidents, captains of industry, and wealthy American women, simply put female hysterics to bed and fed them excessively, believing sheer boredom would drive them back into dutiful health. The nineteenth century's blooming love for the Machine found expression in the use of mechanical devices: "ovary compressors"; coal-fired steam-powered pelvic manipulators; and electromechanical vibrators, including the enormous "Chattanooga Vibrator" (circa 1904), which thundered over prone patients, seeking a cure in one orgasmic release. Science, in the early decades of this century, was a strange amalgam of wisdom and silliness, triumph, experimentation, cruelty, progress, and naiveté. What can seem to us, a century later, a weirdly irreconcilable combination of absurdity and logic was simply then the temper of the times.

What to do about this bewildering plague? Advice poured in from all over the country to the White House, the office of Surgeon General Blue, local authorities, and newspapers.

J.J.C. Elliott, Former Superintendent of Los Angeles' Methodist Hospital, urged the American public:

> Take two pieces of flannel each 12 x 14 inches, sprinkle over one or two of the small packages of wormwood purchased from drug stores usually for ten cents. Lay the other over the sprinkled wormwood and stitch around the edges and quilt them across each way so the wormwood may be held evenly over the entire bag. Place one of these bags in vinegar and place the bag over the chest of the patient, covering the flannel with bed clothing.

Joseph Peloquin of Leavenworth, Kansas, suggested, "Rinse the mouth with lime water, inhale hot water and turpentine fumes." Mrs. Julia Gibson of Pasadena, California, suggested saturating a small rag in alcohol and chloroform and wedging it between one's teeth. Dr. Alexander B. Leeds of Chickasha, Oklahoma, suggested removing one's teeth and tonsils. A citizen from Amarillo, Texas, offered the advice of an "old Mexican man": deeply inhale the acrid smoke of burning straw, hay, or corn cobs. Influenza could also be cured by fondling "sacred pebbles" from a shrine in Kyoshu, Japan. North Carolinians were encouraged to sprinkle sulfur in their shoes, tie sliced fresh cucumbers to their ankles, and carry a potato in each pocket. Others wore necklaces of chicken feathers. Still others kept an ace of diamonds in their left shoe. Some rubbed vinegar over their face while chanting:

> Sour, sour, vinegar-V;
> Keep the sickness off'n me.

In South Chicago, a cobra writhing to the flute of a turbaned snake-charmer coaxed the curious towards bottles of "Spanish Influenza Remedy." In Kwangji, Korea, influenza victims were bludgeoned with clubs "to expel the evil spirit." Major Alfred Friedlander of Camp Sherman, Ohio, was overwhelmed with telegrams suggesting that shotguns placed beneath sickbeds would "draw out" the fever because of the magnetism of the metal. Astrologers were a busy bunch. Perhaps the planet Jupiter was showering Earth with sinister microorganisms. Perhaps the culprit was a disruption of normal astrological geometry: the un-synchronized "vibrations" of Saturn and Neptune, which had been unnaturally occupying the sign of Leo for two years. All over the world, people blamed the weather. Was the culprit Britain's east wind? A humid Swiss fog? Canada's wet summer? Europe's hot, rainless summer? The dry air in Germany?

Chicago's Health Commissioner Robertson declared, "It is our duty to keep the people from fear. For my part, let the people wear a rabbit's foot on a watch chain if they want." But as the epidemic spread, even a lucky rabbit's foot could not help.

> I had a little bird
> And its name was Enza
> I opened the window and
> In-flew-enza.

"In flew Enza?" The Spanish Lady was more like a raptor

than a little bird. Established on both coasts, she began infil-trating towns all across America. She could not be denied, dis-believed, or wished away.

In the tiny hamlet of Meadow, Utah, Lee Reay and his family apprehensively watched the mysterious plague move closer. The *Desert News* was reporting from Salt Lake City that influenza had reached Brigham Young's city. The plague was moving south, along the county highway. He remembers:

> The next thing we knew it was in Nephi and then it was in Fillmore. We were next, just eight miles down the road. It kept coming closer. We told our relatives to stay away. We didn't want visitors of any kind. We didn't want anyone bringing the plague to Meadow.

The town of Meadow organized. Lee Reay's father was elected Health Officer.

> We had never had a health officer before, but we thought we needed one now. So my father, William H. Reay, became Meadow's Health Officer. The first thing Dad did was to tack up signs at the city limits. He hung signs on the northern and southern ends of the only road that ran through Meadow, say-ing, "This Town is Quarantined. Do Not Stop." After that, no-body stopped in Meadow.
>
> But the disease came anyway. We didn't know how it got here. Then, when the mailman got sick, we realized the mail-man had brought the plague to Meadow.

On September 9, the flu-ridden troopship *Leviathan* arrived in New York. Ambulances idled at the dock. One of the scores of sick rushed to area hospitals was an Assistant Secretary of the Navy, a young man suffering from double pneumonia, Franklin Delano Roosevelt. Prince Axel of Denmark, another of the ship's passengers, had avoided the scourge, he claimed, by locking himself in his cabin and downing his prophylactic of choice—whiskey.

The American public confronted a disconcerting fact. America's uniformed "protectors" had become a clear and obvious source of danger. Whether troopship or troop-train, army camp or naval station, the nation's military was engulfed in flu. Sailors, especially—America's "Jackies"—were fueling the epidemic's firestorm spread. On September 7, Jackies from Boston introduced influenza to Philadelphia. Three days later, sailors from Philadelphia brought the flu to Quebec. At the Great Lakes Naval Training Station, thirty miles north of Chicago, influenza appeared on September 11. A week later, twenty-six hundred Jackies were sick. A quarantine was imposed, but it was too late. Influenza had reached Chicago, the heart of the Midwest and the nerve center of the nation's railroads. Soon, the Great Lakes Naval Training Station, the destination of Nurse Josie Mabel Brown, counted eleven thousand ill. In Detroit, Health Commissioner, J.W. Inches informed the army and navy his city was "off-limits" to military personnel. Only personnel on critical military business and in perfect health, as confirmed in writing by a superior officer, would be allowed into the city. Almost immediately, Inches' directive was rendered irrelevant. Thousands in Detroit were sick.

What sailors began, soldiers often completed. Troops from Texas introduced influenza to Kentucky when their train paused in Bowling Green. A soldier on leave from Camp Forest, Georgia brought the flu to Elco, Illinois (population 236). The soldier, suffering a "cold," infected his fiancee, his cousin, and the daughter of Elco's postmaster. Within days, influenza had reached every household in Elco.

At military facilities across America, barracks were being converted into contagion wards. Buglers were failing to sound reveille. At Camp Grant, Illinois, 10,713 soldiers were sick; at Camp Dodge, Iowa, 8,000; at Camp Meade, Maryland, 11,000; in Norfolk, Virginia, 5,000. Nevertheless, the massive wartime effort continued. On September 17, Jackies from Philadelphia arrived in the Puget Sound Naval Yard, outside of Seattle. Immediately, 173 local sailors fell ill. The camp's chief medical officer was unfazed. He declared: "Now that the glamour of the early days of Spain cannot be cast about the influenza, it will be compelled to pass on its way unhonored and unsung." Three days later, Puget Sound's National Guard Infantry held a festive public review. Ten thousand civilians jammed the station. By September 25, influenza was epidemic in Seattle.

> Were the men and women in positions of authority in the western states, especially in the field of public health, all incompetent? Again, the answer is no, just as it was east of the Mississippi. Very few health officers and no communities as a whole really appreciated the devastation the pandemic could wreak until experiencing it. Spanish influenza was just too new, too unprecedented, and it moved faster than the human mind could assimilate the news of it.
>
> —Alfred Crosby, Historian

On the night of September 27, Vermont's Fifty-Seventh Pioneer division set out on a march to join their fellow doughboys on the troopship *Leviathan*. Men began falling out of ranks, collapsing in the dirt.

> The column was halted and the camp surgeon was summoned. The examination showed that the dreaded influenza had hit us. Although many men had fallen out, we were ordered to resume the march. We went forward up and up over the winding

moonlit road leading to Alpine Landing on the Hudson where ferry boats were waiting to take us to Hoboken.

The victims of the epidemic fell on either side of the road, unable to carry their heavy packs. Some threw their equipment away and with determination tried to keep up with their comrades. Army trucks and ambulances, following, picked up those who had fallen.

—Colonel E.W. Gibson

In the first week of October, all schools in Boston were closed. Seven-year-old Francis Russell escaped the long reach of his teacher, Miss Sykes. He later recalled:

> For us it was pure joy in that abounding weather to be free of the third grade and the Palmer Method and the multiplication tables and Miss Sykes and her harmonica. The early mornings turned frosty, blackening the marigolds, but the afternoons were warm and sun-drenched and golden, heavy with cricket sounds, light as milkweed down. By Collins' Pond the witch hazel was in bloom, the lemon-yellow filaments crisscrossed against the bare branches. On the Hill, on such bright days, we lost ourselves in the immediacy of the timeless present, as free to wander as any coma of milkweed.

In his office in Washington D.C., just down the hall from Surgeon General Rupert Blue, epidemiologist Victor Vaughan was working late. Statistics were coming in from all over the world. At lightening-bolt speed, the epidemic was racing across the globe, through the world's population of nearly two billion people. The numbers were terrifying. In India alone, millions were already dying.

Vaughan poured over the masses of statistics, trying to understand this bewildering disease, find the truth hiding within the numbers. He had already discovered certain tendencies. "City dwellers acquire some degree of immunity because they live in an atmosphere bearing infections. Country boys are more highly susceptible." Native Americans, who tended to live in rural areas, were suffering hideously, dying at a rate four times higher than that of people in large cities. But blacks, usually more vulnerable to respiratory diseases than whites, had a lower death rate. Strange. Tragically, pregnant women were being hit disproportionately hard, suffocating quickly as their fluid-filled lungs swelled into their cramped thorax. In one town in New Hampshire, thirty-six young mothers had already died.

Finally, the numbers were telling Vaughan what, by now, nearly everyone knew. Ordinarily, influenza killed only the very young and the very old. But this disease had a different target. "Like war," Vaughan wrote, "[Spanish influenza] kills young, vigorous, robust adults."

In Dorchester, Francis Russell and his friend Eliot Dodds watched as Everett Nudd, a grim, sulky-faced boy, cut across a field and headed down the Hollow toward New Calvary cemetery. "Sissy, sissy," Eliot cried out, taunting Everett. Then, strangely curious, Francis and Eliot sprinted across the grass and fell into step behind him, following Everett down the road toward the cemetery. Everett spun on his heel. "Want to come along?" he goaded. "Want to come watch funerals? I do it every day." Francis had never been to a funeral. The idea terrified him, but neither he nor Eliot could turn back.

> We wandered down the main path past the brown and gray stone monuments, past carved crosses and sacred hearts and triumphant stone angels with impassive granite wings. Then

the path ended at a dump, and Everett turned right through a thicket of ground oak and speckled alder, holding up his hand in warning. A funeral was going on directly below us. Around the raw earth of an open grave a group of mourners was huddled together like a flock of bedraggled starlings. The fumed oak coffin had been set beside the grave, and a priest in a biretta stood at its head, even as we looked down, making the sign of the cross over it. Then the others began to file past and some of them stopped to pick up a bit of earth which they scattered on the coffin. Just behind them two workmen appeared with ropes fastened in a sling. A heavy-built man with white hair and florid features stopped at the grave's edge, shook the damp clay from his fingers, then glanced up to see us peering through the alder bushes. "Get out of here, you!" he shouted, his face turning scarlet. "Get out!"

The boys ducked into the bushes. But Everett tugged on Francis' shirt. He had something more to tell him. Weary gravediggers, hopelessly behind, were simply dumping out the bodies when no one was looking and reusing the coffins. The boys emerged from the bushes beside yet another open grave.

A grave digger had just climbed out and stood with his shovel beside him, lighting his pipe. He was an old Italian with a drooping mustache, wearing a shapeless felt hat with a turned-down brim. The grave digger stared at us with shrewd, uncomprehending eyes, then took his pipe out of his mouth and spat again. "Ah, you boys-a go-onna home," he said thickly. "You no playa here. Go-onna home."

Francis fled. He raced home, out of breath, furious, distraught. Even the lights of home, the glow in the kitchen where his mother was making dinner, could not reassure him.

Seeing the lights, thinking of the afternoon, in that bare instant I became aware of time. I knew then that life was not a perpetual present, and that even tomorrow would be part of the past, and that for all my days and years to come I too must one day die. I pushed the relentless thought aside, knowing even as I did...I should never again be wholly free of it.

Chapter 4

Pandemic

Louis Brownlow of Washington, D.C., was worried. Like New York's Royal Copeland, Brownlow was a city commissioner, but Brownlow was Copeland's opposite in temperament and outlook. On October 2, 1918, Brownlow was informed that a single Washington hospital had admitted forty patients with "la grippe." Brownlow was aware of the situation in New England; just the day before, 202 Bostonians had died of influenza. Immediately, Brownlow phoned his city coroner. "Ramsay," he said, "be prepared for the worst." The Spanish Lady, Brownlow realized, was at the gates of his city. Immediately Brownlow did everything he could. He closed schools, theaters, pool halls, and bars. He set up nursing centers in empty school buildings, and transformed a store on F Street into an emergency hospital under the supervision of a Public Health Service epidemiologist, Dr. James P. Leake. Brownlow limited store hours and banned public gatherings. Cinemas went dark. The names in the marquees disappeared. No more "Laughing Bill Hyde" with Will Rogers. No more Dorothy Gish in "Battling Jane." The final curtain fell on *Frolics of the Night: Flo-Flo and her Perfect Thirty-Six Chorus* at the National Burlesque. Even President Woodrow Wilson would have to forego his weekly diversion, vaudeville at the B.F. Keith's Theater. The capital shut down.

Louis Brownlow acted swiftly and he acted alone. He had no choice. D.C.'s two other city commissioners were sick with influenza. Brownlow phoned Washington's elite. A garage along posh Embassy Row was transformed into the headquarters of a Motor Ambulance Corps. Model T trucks and donated, chauffeur-driven limousines roared to life. The Motor Corps sped through the city, bringing soup and blankets to the stricken and removing the deathly ill to Dr. Leake's hospital. Other eminent Washingtonians voiced their support. Dr. Noble P. Barnes, publicly exhorted, "Persons at large sneezing and coughing should be treated as a dangerous menace to the community, properly fined, imprisoned, and compelled to wear masks until they are educated out of that 'Gesundheit!' and 'God Bless You' rot." The Red Cross distributed thousands of gauze face masks. Ads admonished the public:

> Obey the laws
> And wear the gauze
> Protect your jaws
> From septic paws.

But neither catchy jingles, nor the exhortations of Noble Barnes, nor Louis Brownlow's determined closures could prevent the spread of the disease. The number of ill quickly soared above ten thousand. Hundreds of policemen and trolley drivers fell sick. So many firemen were ill that, according to D.C.'s Fire Marshall: "The whole city'd burn to the ground if a fire ever got started." The Federal government was becoming crippled. Courts recessed indefinitely. Half of the employees at Herbert Hoover's Food Administration were sick. What little staff remained in the Departments of State, War, and Navy was "aired" for twenty minutes each day—marched outside and asked to breathe deeply. Congress closed its public galleries. Still, the contagion spread. W. E. Turton, a clerk in the Vital Statistics Bureau, died, even as he poured over Washington's disturbing mortality tables. The *Wash-*

ington Evening Star began publishing a column, "Prominent People Who Have Died of Influenza."

Washington was engulfed in disease. No one felt the terrifying presence of the plague more than six-year-old Bill Sardo. Bill Sardo's family operated a Washington funeral home. In Bill's house, life had literally become invaded by death. Caskets were everywhere. People were laid out in the living room, the dining room, and the hallways. Bill assembled caskets in the basement morgue. He remembers: "I was constantly afraid. I would walk through rows and rows of caskets, seeing names, people I knew. Entire families were dying. The dead were everywhere."

The second week of October brought no relief. Terrified Washingtonians lashed out at Brownlow. Pastors wanted their churches reopened. Brownlow was condemned by the District Pastors' Federation; an esteemed Presbyterian minister, Dr. Wallace Radcliffe, urged, "It is necessary that the spiritual dynamo be kept running at full speed." Dr. H.S. Mustard, a Public Health Service epidemiologist and specialist in malaria control, was appointed D.C.'s "Health Czar." Mustard confronted Brownlow, saying, "If we don't keep Washington going now, there won't be any France!" Brownlow's measures, Mustard claimed, "weren't enough." One out of every three people in the nation's capital was wearing face masks, masks which were, Mustard contended, "maybe as effective as fish nets against flies." Louis Brownlow was not intimidated; he had found an ally. Brownlow and Mustard declared Washington a "sanitary zone." They divided the city into four self-contained units. Separate medical, nursing, and volunteer staffs would serve each district. A new law decreed that "No person shall knowingly expose himself or any other persons, or if he has the power and authority to prevent, permit any other person to be exposed to infection of epidemic influenza."

In Washington, it was now a crime to ("knowingly") transmit

influenza. It was also criminal for the sick to venture out in public. Fines were a hefty fifty dollars and up.

Every hospital bed in the nation's capital was full. At George Washington University Hospital, not one nurse remained standing. In Garfield Hospital and Leake's emergency hospital, influenza patients spilled out of crammed rooms into equally-crowded hallways. Leake despaired: "The only way we could find room for the sick was to have undertakers waiting at the back door, ready to remove bodies as fast as people died. The living came in one door and the dead went out the other." Louis Brownlow became obsessed with the dead. At nearby Camp Humphreys, five thousand soldiers were sick with influenza. The camp's chief medical officer, Lieutenant Colonel Charles E. Doerr, had died. Still, Brownlow begged fifty soldiers from Camp Humphreys to dig graves for Washingtonians. The soldiers were ordered to dig grave after grave, as fast as they could. But there were no coffins for the graves. Coffins had become as rare as black pearls and nearly as priceless. Some morticians, responding to the mercenary laws of supply and demand, were price-gouging. A Washington official proclaimed, "Charging high prices for coffins in this direful time is nothing short of ghoulish in spirit and unpatriotic to the point of treason." But Brownlow himself resorted to stealing. Tipped off that two carloads of coffins destined for Pittsburgh had paused in the Potomac freight yards, Brownlow simply hijacked the shipment. The coffins were removed to the playground of Central High School and placed under armed guard.

Louis Brownlow put out a desperate call for volunteers. His plea reached Mrs. Herbert Hoover, as well as "Flo-Flo and her Perfect Thirty-Six." The Motor Ambulance Corps became reinforced by Mrs. Fairchild's Red Cross Motor Corps, which cruised the city night and day, seeking the sick and the dead. A young teacher, Esther Jonas, converted the empty classrooms of Wilson Normal School into a soup kitchen, serving 350 meals a day to medical personnel and volunteers. Jonas witnessed examples of "great courage" and "great cowardice":

> So many landlords and landladies abandoned their tenants, leaving them ill and in atrocious condition. The volunteers, however, were wonderful. They came to my kitchen in great numbers. One old lady said she couldn't do anything except wash dishes. And wash dishes she did, mountains of dishes.

One afternoon, Louis Brownlow received a telephone call from a sobbing woman. She shared a room with three other girls. Two of the girls were dead, she said; the third was dying. She was the only one who was well. Brownlow was nursing his wife (also sick with the flu). He called the police and asked them to hurry over. A few hours later, a police sergeant called Brownlow back with the concise report: "Four girls dead."

In another part of the nation's capital, a volunteer nurse knocked on a door. She heard a rasping "Come in, come in." She entered. To her horror, only a pet parrot remained alive in the house. The nurse fled, the parrot's shrill, macabre invitation still echoing in her ears.

In Macon, Georgia, the shadow of the sugar magnolias had lengthened. Crows reeled across fields of goldenrod.

> I knew we were in trouble when my mother became sick. I knew it from my child's eye and my child's eye was five years old. I wanted to get in bed with her, but it wasn't allowed; they didn't want me to get sick. So they brought a little bed into her room for me. Still, I tossed and turned. I wanted to be in bed with her. Finally, she said, "Climb in with me, Katherine."
>
> —Katherine Guyler

The pain began behind Katherine's eyes. Pain spread quickly down her body, to her chest, her belly, her legs. Her teeth chattered. Katherine felt a scalding Georgia heat. A screen door slammed in the wind. Hot wind stirred the parched corn. Grasshoppers sizzled across the red earth. Someone was rubbing her chest. "Open your mouth," a voice said.

> I was in so much pain, my father sent for Dr. Clark. We had one doctor in Macon and he had only one medicine and it was called Dr. Clark's Medicine. To this day, I don't know what was in it, but no matter what you had, you got Dr. Clark's Medicine and then you prayed for the best.

In New Haven, Connecticut, John Deleno continued to play on the coffins stacked outside the neighborhood mortuary.

> One day, my three best buddies didn't come out of their houses in the morning. I realized no one in our neighborhood was visiting each other. No one was passing around food, talking on the street. Everyone was staying inside. Still, every morning, I went to my buddies' houses. I knocked on the door and waited for them to come out and play.

In 1918, San Francisco, California, was a modest metropolis of 550,000. Like many American cities, San Francisco was swollen with recent immigrants (especially Italians and Chinese), and home as well to a number of military installations. On September 21, the chief of San Francisco's Board of Health, Dr. William Hassler, urged that precautions be taken to protect the city from the flu. Quarantines were imposed at the Yerba Buena Island Naval Training Station and other Bay Area naval installations. Hassler was a well-known city official, both celebrated and notorious. Immediately after the 1906 earthquake, he had established a births and deaths registry on the porch of his house; he and Rupert Blue had guided the city through several cycles of bubonic plague. This time, however, the seasoned Hassler vacillated. He reversed himself, saying he doubted influenza would reach San Francisco after all.

Talk of further quarantines or closures was suspended. A myriad of festive public gatherings commenced. On September 28, the Fourth Liberty Loan Drive was inaugurated. Ten thousand paraded down Market Street, displaying an effigy of Kaiser Wilhelm nailed inside an open coffin. Twenty-five thousand San Franciscans joined in a patriotic "community sing." Mary Pickford addressed thousands at a rally at the Bethlehem Shipbuilding Corporation. On October 6, 150,000 massed in Golden Gate Park and formed into columns of marchers. Loudspeakers blared, "Yours will be the greatest motion picture ever made, for it is to take your smile and your kiss to your soldiers over there." Movie cameras began rolling. For three hours, patriotic marchers filed past, blowing kisses at the celluloid.

A few days later, French tenor Lucien Muratore sang the "Star Spangled Banner" and "La Marseillaise" to a crowd of fifty thousand from the steps of the Chronicle Building. In the middle of the national anthem, an ambulance wailed; the throng parted to let the vehicle pass.

A week later, San Francisco was engulfed in flu.

In Royal Copeland's New York, 3,077 residents fell sick with influenza in a single day. At Columbia Presbyterian Hospital, Dr. Albert Lamb reported droves of incoming patients: "They're blue as huckleberries and spitting blood."

New York's Bellevue Hospital was packed. People were dying

not just in beds and on stretchers and cots, but also on the floor of crowded corridors. In jammed pediatric wards, sick children languished three to a bed. In the hospital basement, terrified laundresses panicked and fled, abandoning their washtubs. At Columbia Presbyterian Hospital, any semblance of routine had been abandoned. Dorothy Deming, a student nurse, later recalled:

> There were no more formal "doctors' rounds," neither for the attending physicians nor for the medical students. Doctors came and went at all hours, calling for a nurse only when giving an order or needing help. It was quite usual to see a haggard doctor come in long after midnight to make a last examination of his patient before staggering home to bed.

Often, sadness overwhelmed Deming and her friend, another nurse, also named Dorothy.

> Until the epidemic, death had seemed kindly, coming to the very old, the incurably suffering, or striking suddenly without the knowledge of its victims. Now, we saw death clutch cruelly and ruthlessly at vigorous, well-muscled young women in the prime of life. Flu dulled their resistance, choked their lungs, swamped their hearts. . . . There was nothing but sadness and horror to this senseless waste of human life.
>
> Many a morning, after working hard over a patient, Dorothy [Deming's friend] and I bore the grim task of trying to find words of comfort for dazed parents, husbands and children. One dawn—a glorious morning with rose-colored clouds above the gray buildings across the street—after a particularly sad death, I knew the tears I had been shedding inwardly must find outlet. I rushed to the linen closet, always our place of refuge, and there ahead of me was Dorothy, sobbing her heart out.

The Atlantic Division of the Red Cross met in emergency session. Thirty-one of their 170 nurses were sick with flu. New York policemen, firemen, trolley drivers, telephone operators, and garbage collectors were ill and morticians and cemetery workers were overwhelmed. War production faltered: Staten Island's naval shipyards were experiencing a 40 percent absenteeism. Exhausted public health workers, combing the boroughs, entered upon nightmarish scenes. In rank, crowded tenements, the dead lay shoulder to shoulder with the dying. Everywhere: the sobs of feverish children, the sound of hacking coughs, moans, and whimpers. And on the street the melancholy sound of funeral processions. The slow creak of carriage wheels. The clip-clop of horses' hooves.

Still, New York's optimistic Copeland refused to despair. He also refused to close schools or theaters. "I'm keeping my theaters in as good condition as my wife keeps our home," he told the press. "And I can vouch that is perfectly sanitary." The epidemic, he said, was not "serious." He preferred to call it "widespread." On the day of Copeland's decision, 354 New Yorkers died of influenza. The mayor ordered city engineers to start digging graves.

By now, all over the world millions were sick. People in Hong Kong were suffering "the-too-muchee-hot sickness"; Hungarians, "The Black Whip"; the Japanese, "wrestler's fever"; and the Persians, "the disease of the wind." Three quarters of Manila's dock workers were incapacitated with "*trancazo*," "a blow from a heavy stick." In Switzerland, "the coquette" continued her unscrupulous solicitation of victims. Siam was shaking with "*Kai Wat Yai*," "the Great Cold Fever." With caprice and deadly accuracy, the Spanish Lady played her role again and again. The globe had truly become her stage.

In Rio de Janeiro, two hundred thousand were sick; in the

Black Sea port of Odessa, seventh-five thousand. In Russia's Stalag Josefstadt, prisoners of war who had died of influenza were stacked twenty men high, then covered in snow. In Tangier, North Africa, hearses became mired in the muddy, jammed roads leading to the city's cemeteries. The London *Times* reported from Barcelona:

> The newspapers give the death toll from the disease as three hundred a day, the Civil Governor states it is six hundred a day, and the medical men with whom I have spoken say it cannot be less than twelve hundred a day.
>
> In places there is panic; the theaters, music halls, and public restaurants are more than half empty, dancing is forbidden, and the people go about inhaling eucalyptol, creosote, or whatever the prevalent essential oil may be. Funerals are working day and night and coffins are almost unobtainable.

In Cape Town, South Africa, where tens of thousands were sick, a friend asked Dr. Frederick Willmot, Assistant Medical Officer of Health, "Are we going to be wiped out?" Willmot replied, "I'll tell you what I wouldn't tell any other man in the Union. For the first time in my life I'm panicky, and I believe we are."

On the South Pacific island of Fiji, both natives and whites were "dying like flies." Alick Rea, of the Colonial Sugar Refining Company, reported home to Sydney, Australia:

> For a full week, I was the only person moving about in this particular district. Everything was still and quiet... except for the hacking cough of the unfortunates who had developed pneumonia as a complication. Deaths occurred so quickly that it was only with the greatest difficulty that sepulture could be given to the remains.
>
> The epidemic, strangely enough, has hit hard among car-

penters, and there is only one man left who can make coffins.
As it is not certain how long this man will last, he is making
full use of his time getting coffins ready.

In Samoa, eight thousand islanders were dead. New Zealanders
lent a hand. The *Sydney Daily Telegraph* reported:

> At one time, 80 or 90 percent of the [Samoan] people were
> lying helpless, many died from starvation who might probably
> have recovered, for even when rice, milk, and other items were
> sent out and delivered, the survivors were too weak to prepare
> and apportion the food. In the small town of Apia and its en-
> virons, nearly seven hundred were buried.
>
> The New Zealand troopers with their motor-trucks are
> doing wonderful service day after day gathering up the dead,
> who are simply lifted out of their houses as they lie on their
> sleeping-mats. The mats are wrapped around them, and they
> are deposited in one great pit at Vaimea after it was found im-
> possible to get laborers to dig individual graves. There are no
> mourners, there is no ceremony. As fast as the different
> motor-trucks come, the bodies are placed in the pit by heroic
> workers, many of whom are quite unfit and who have to quit
> as they themselves become infected. Most of the great chiefs
> of Samoa have been buried.

Examples of compassion and cooperation among racial and
ethnic groups existed alongside their opposite, less charitable
extreme. Terrified and baffled, many continued to assign blame.
The Poles called the malady "The Bolshevik Disease." Russians
blamed nomadic Kirghiz tribesmen. Germans blamed the one
hundred thousand Chinese imported to dig trenches for the
war. As influenza ravaged Argentina, the Spanish dish *paella*
was banned from restaurant menus. In anti-Semitic Warsaw,

sanitarians called the Jewish ghetto: "a particular enemy of order and cleanliness." Some hospitals in West Africa refused to treat blacks. In Montreal, the *Gazette* blithely announced, "No Panic Except Amongst Orientals."

Perhaps the greatest horror was occurring in India. All over India, immense mountains of bodies were rising beside fiery ghats. Oozing through the slums of Calcutta, the Hooghly River was "choked with bodies." The Associated Press reported:

> Streets and lanes of India's cities are littered with the dead. Hospitals are so choked, it is impossible to remove the dead to make room for the dying. Burning ghats and burial grounds are literally piled with corpses.

Despite the efforts to quarantine the town, the postman had delivered the "phantom" to Meadow, Utah. Lee Reay's entire family fell sick, including Lee and his father, William Reay, Meadow's Health Officer. As he slowly recuperated, Lee's father traveled the town, checking on his neighbors. Lee Reay recalls:

> My father needed to find out which families had the sickness, so he rode from farm to farm on his horse. He would shout in his big, strong voice, "Is everybody okay in there?" And they would either reply, "Yes, we're okay," or, "We need help." Then he would ask, "What kind of help do you need?"—"We need medicine" or "We need help milking our cows" or "We need someone to do our chores." Then Dad would get help. But first, he'd nail a big yellow sign on the front gate which said, "This House Is Quarantined. Do Not Enter."
>
> Nobody was visiting anyone in Meadow. We were all too scared. Meadow was a Mormon town and we all helped each other, that was part of our religion. But we wanted to help each

other from a distance. The Ladies Relief Society brought food and water to sick families. They'd leave it on the doorstep, then run away. Everyone wore a handkerchief over their face—a big, red bandanna like the cowboys wore. Although I was just a boy, I helped, too. I harvested our garden and I'd put beets, carrots, and other produce in a bucket. I'd tie a red bandanna around my face, put the bucket on the front step of a house, knock on the door, and run. Then I'd watch from the gate to make sure somebody crawled to the door to get the food. I also milked cows. Everyone in Meadow had cows and they had to be milked, morning and night. I was a good milker, so I milked cows for a half dozen families. I also fed the chickens and the pigs.

On a balmy September day, the fishing schooner *Leverna* left Gloucester, Massachusetts. She returned a few days later without a single halibut, but with twenty-three fishermen, her entire crew, sick with influenza. A Japanese vessel, the *Shensi Maru*, limped into a U.S. Naval Station in the Azores, captain and crew delirious, several men dead. For days, the *Shensi Maru* had been adrift in the Atlantic. Spanish influenza traveled across the world on trucks and trains, by car and by foot, but ships had become the deadliest places in the world to get sick and the swiftest, surest way to spread the contagion. The overstuffed troopships crisscrossing the Atlantic were increasingly lethal. Whether converted passenger vessels or military men-of-war, America's troopships were meeting the demands of General Pershing and French Marshal Foch by increasing capacity by half and then some. Called "intensive loading," rather then the more accurate "fifty percent overload," overcrowding, by whatever name, was proving ideal for the proliferation of an illness borne by a sneeze.

War is a game of cat and mouse, strategy and hunches. Neither Pershing nor Foch nor Woodrow Wilson knew what German commander Erich von Ludendorff knew. Ludendorff was a realist; by late September, he realized the war had been lost. Since August 8's "Black Day," when Foch's Amiens offensive had devastated German forces south of the Somme (killing twenty thousand Germans in five days), the Kaiser's troops had been wearily, quietly surrendering to the Allies. On September 29, Ludendorff asked that a new German government begin armistice negotiations with the Allies. He recorded bitterly:

> I have asked His Majesty to bring those people into the government who are largely responsible that things have turned out as they have. We shall therefore see these gentlemen enter the ministries, and they must now make the peace which has to be made. They must now eat the soup they have ladled out to us.

On the other side of Europe's barbed trenches, Allied Commander Foch sensed victory was within reach. The war, however, had not been won. Victory depended on American doughboys. In the fall of 1918, a half million doughboys crossed the Atlantic. Not a single troopship was sunk by a German U-boat. Still, a much deadlier enemy loomed. On September 21, the U.S.S. *Yacona* left New London, Connecticut, for Nova Scotia. By Boston, she could go no further; 80 of the 96 on board were sick. The man-of-war U.S.S. *Pittsburgh* docked in flu-ridden Rio de Janeiro; 647 sailors took sick and 58 died, dozens more than embalmers could handle. Coffins were carried on donkey carts through Rio's sweltering streets to San Francisco Xavier Cemetery.

On October 12, the Navy canceled the directive that men who died at sea be returned home. Sailors and soldiers were to be buried in local ports or shrouded in the American flag and released overboard. In early October, influenza provoked one of the deadliest naval accidents of the war. A flu-ridden convoy became hopelessly lost in a gale off the coast of Northern Ireland. Crippled by crews so sick with influenza that orders became as compromised and unclear as visibility, the *Kashmir* rammed into the side of the *Otranto*. The *Otranto's* boilers exploded. Steam shot heavenward. The ship began sinking, sending 431 sailors into the frigid waters of the North Atlantic. The captain of a nearby vessel, Lieutenant-Commander Francis Craven, R.N., watched helplessly as the *Otranto's* smiling captain waved calmly on the sinking deck, a doomed bugler warbled "Abandon ship," and a sailor, half-buried in charred bodies, laughed hysterically.

Cables from Brest, France, tersely announced that American convoys were arriving with overwhelming numbers of sick and dead. Ninety-seven of the *President Grant's* human cargo arrived dead. On October 7, the *Leviathan*, America's mightiest transport, arrived in Brest with an equivalent number of corpses. How could this happen on the *Leviathan*? The *Leviathan* was a whale of a ship, carrying upwards of twelve thousand at a time, zipping across the Atlantic at a daunting twelve knots an hour. The ship was, in fact, German. The *"Vaterland"* was cruising past America when war broke out. Forced to seek sanctuary in the home of her eventual enemy, she was commandeered by the United States in 1917 and renamed after the behemoths of the oceans. But the *Leviathan's* latest round-trip, which ended in Brest on October 7, had been ill-fated from the start. Arriving in New York on September 9, she had delivered scores of sick, including a young Assistant Secretary of the Navy, Franklin Delano Roosevelt, to area hospitals. Marching to meet her, Vermont's Fifty-seventh Pioneer Infantry had seen countless soldiers fall from their ranks on the moonlit road to the Hudson River. Although men who showed obvious signs of illness had been left behind in New York, seven hundred fell sick on the *Leviathan* after only a single day at sea. The hospital was crammed. Stricken soldiers languished all over the ship. The healthy were "quarantined"—shuffled from port side to starboard and back again, then down into unventilated catacombs (considered unfit for human habitation) or onto heaving, wave-lashed decks. The chaotic shuffle ended as the number of sick swelled above two thousand and any attempts at quarantine became impossible. Physicians, nurses, and the ship's chief surgeon fell ill. A ghoulish problem arose: how to identify the delirious and the dead. Inexplicably, hundreds of the soldiers' dogtags were utterly blank. The *Leviathan's* Colonel Gibson later wrote:

> The conditions cannot be visualized by anyone who has not actually seen them. Pools of blood from severe nasal hemorrhages of many patients were scattered throughout the compartments, and the attendants were powerless to escape tracking through the mess, because of the narrow passages between the bunks. The decks became wet and slippery, groans and cries of the terrified added to the confusion of the applicants clamoring for treatment, and altogether a true inferno reigned supreme.

Orderlies picked among the dying for the dead. The *Leviathan's* War Diary recorded: "small force of embalmers impossible to keep up with rate of dying—impossible to embalm bodies fast enough—signs of decomposing starting in some of them." When the vessel arrived in France, 969 influenza victims were taken to Brest's already-crammed hospitals. For two hundred doughboys, the Atlantic journey on America's mightiest troopship ended in a French cemetery in Lambezellec.

Similar stories were being told all across the world's oceans. On the flu-ravaged *Briton*, Private Robert James Wallace rocked for twelve days on a salty, heaving deck, feverishly drifting in and out of consciousness. One morning, he was moved suddenly inside— to a room which, in the peacetime past, had served as a saloon. A nurse appeared. She asked if he wanted her to wash his feet. Fifty years later, Robert Wallace recalled: "That gentle washing of my feet with her soft soapy hands engraved a memory in my mind

which I shall record in Heaven when I get there." Wallace passed
out. He awoke. A sick soldier was weakly nudging his arm. The
man begged for water. Wallace was too sick to do anything but
call. Over and over, he feebly called for water, but neither his
angel nor a medic appeared. Finally, the thirsty man whispered,
"Don't bother anymore." Wallace continued calling. "I won't
need it," the thirsty man said. The next morning, when medics finally arrived, the soldier was dead. According to Wallace, "he had
rolled—in some final, dim, instinctual effort to gain protection—
under the settee. They carried him out for burial."

In Lincoln, Illinois, William Maxwell's mother was expecting
a baby. The Maxwells had decided to have the baby in Bloomington at a large city hospital. William and his brother were sent
to stay with their aunt and uncle. The house was dark and
gloomy. In the dining room was a vase of peacock feathers, har-
bingers, William knew, of bad luck.

> My aunt and uncle were narrow-minded, church-going people.
> My brother and I were very uncomfortable being in their
> house. I can best suggest the quality of the house by saying in
> the living room there was a framed photograph of my grand-
> father in his coffin. There were also a lot of things we were not
> allowed to play with. Right after we arrived, I fell sick. I was a
> skinny little boy with an enormous appetite, but just as my
> plate was put in front of me, I felt no desire for food. My aunt
> had cooked turkey with stuffing, everything I enjoyed, cran-
> berries and so forth, but I looked at it and all I could say was,
> "I don't feel hungry." At the same time I didn't feel hungry, I
> also had a keen sense of grief that I wasn't going to get to enjoy
> dinner. My aunt put her hand my forehead. I had a high fever.
> She took me upstairs and put me to bed in my uncle's office.

The office had a table in it, a desk, a typewriter, photographs of my ancestors, all the agents of our fire insurance company. There was nothing to comfort or reassure a little boy in that room. It was bleak in the extreme.

I think what happened was that I slept and slept and slept and slept. Although I didn't really like my aunt and uncle, they were people you could count on in trouble. A doctor had given them pills, God only knows what. I remember being awakened at intervals during the night and day. If it was night, my aunt would be in a nightgown with her hair in a braid down her back, holding a pill out to me and a glass of water. At other times, it was my uncle.

In Katherine Anne Porter's "Pale Horse, Pale Rider," Miranda has a dream:

Where are my boots and what horse shall I ride? Fiddler or Graylie or Miss Lucy with the long nose and the wicked eye?... I'll take Graylie because he is not afraid of bridges.

Come now, Graylie, she said, taking his bridle, we must outrun Death and the Devil. You are no good for it, she told the other horses standing saddled before the stable gate, among them the horse of the stranger, grey also, with tarnished nose and ears. The stranger swung into his saddle beside her, leaned far towards her and regarded her without meaning, the blank still stare of mindless malice that makes no threats and can bide its time. She drew Graylie around sharply, urged him to run. He leaped the low rose hedge and the narrow ditch beyond, and the dust of the lane flew heavily under his beating hoofs. The stranger rode beside her, easily, lightly, his reins loose in his half-closed hand, straight and elegant in dark shabby garments that flapped upon his bones;

his pale face smiled in an evil trance, he did not glance at her. Ah, I have seen this fellow before, I know this man if I could place him. He is no stranger to me.

On September 26, Massachusetts Senator John Weeks called for a million dollars to fight Spanish influenza. Senator Weeks was himself convalescing from the flu. He told the Senate Appropriations Committee that five members of his family were sick and no bed existed in any hospital for the family maid, who was dying from massive pneumonia. The U.S. Public Health Service displayed a map of the nation, color-coded to indicate the spread of the epidemic. The Eastern Seaboard was still "red hot," including the nation's capital (the Speaker of the House, Champ Cark, was home with the flu). Influenza had spread beyond the nation's military camps, and had reached epidemic proportions in twenty states. On the "safe" side of the Atlantic, 127,975 American soldiers were sick; 3,369 had died. The Public Health Service warned Senators that influenza would continue to spread and thrive in industrial centers. "It is certain that all war projects will be knocked out fifty percent." Henry Cabot Lodge testified: "If the disease is not arrested, it may spread to every part of the country. Already it has affected our munitions plants. Its ravages may be more severe unless we grapple with it now, and we cannot do it without money." In a blunt address, Surgeon General Rupert Blue told Senators that health and relief agencies were overwhelmed with requests for aspirin, quinine, morphine, rubbing alcohol, pajamas, masks, soap, hot water bottles, fly paper, and padded "pneumonia jackets." The Red Cross had authorized $575,000 in emergency funds. The U.S. Public Health Service had *no* funds for epidemic control, however. A million-dollar-appropriation represented a substantial amount—a full one-third of the Public Health Service's annual budget.

The resolution shot through both houses of Congress in two hours without a single dissenter.

In France, General John "Black Jack" Pershing paced on the terrace of Château of Chaumont-en-Bassigny, 160 miles southeast of Paris. For days, the fifty-eight-year-old, four-star general, Commander-in-Chief of the two million American soldiers in France had been, in the words of an aide: "grey with lack of sleep and unceasing strain." He paced continuously, wreathed in the smoke of a *Romeo y Julieta* cigar. A thirty-six year Army veteran, Pershing had faced adversaries like Sitting Bull, Geronimo, and the Mexican revolutionary Francisco "Pancho" Villa. Now, an invisible enemy—the shadowy Spanish Lady—was proving deadlier even than Erich von Ludendorff's dogged German legions. In one week in the Argonne alone, sixteen thousand American soldiers had come down with influenza, joining the seventy thousand already sick. German troops, decimated by influenza's spring wave, seemed, for the moment, immune to this more lethal, fall strain, a strain which was devastating Pershing's fresh American divisions. Still, Marshal Foch continued to pressure Pershing. More doughboys were needed. Only fresh, energetic American troops could smash through the Hindenburg Line and secure an Allied victory. Pershing cabled Washington: "Influenza exists in epidemic form amongst our troops. Request fifteen thousand members of Army Nurse Corps. RUSH RUSH RUSH." Then he cabled for more men. But this time, Pershing's plea hit a stone wall.

The Provost Marshal General of the Army, General Enoch Crowder, had spent much of the month of September charged with the onerous task of identifying and rounding up draft dodgers. Spanish influenza, however, soon eclipsed even the compelling, thorny issue of America's "slackers." Nearly all army camps in the United States were under quarantine. Conditions in Europe were even worse. Only a few weeks earlier, the Chief Surgeon of the Port of New York had declared, "We can't stop this war on account of Spanish or any other kind of influenza." He turned out to be wrong. Influenza now had higher priority than the war. On October 7, Crowder canceled the army's October draft for 142,000 new recruits. An additional draft of 78,000 men, scheduled for late October, was canceled as well.

President Woodrow Wilson faced a crucial and agonizing decision. On October 6, Max, Prince of Baden and Imperial Chancellor of Germany, had appealed to the President to begin negotiations for an armistice. Neither Marshal Foch nor General Pershing nor Wilson himself trusted the efficacy of Max's plea. Germany was in turmoil. Could an imperial ruler guarantee the response of the German people? Was it consistent or even correct for Wilson—democracy's most vocal and eloquent advocate—to deal with a government which was not a government of the people? Like Foch and Pershing, Wilson sensed only a decisive military victory was a truly secure one. On the other hand, the war was fueling the deadly pandemic. To consign fresh recruits to army camps or crowded troopships would mean sending thousands of men to their deaths. A few days earlier, Dr. Victor Heiser, an eminent sanitarian had stated, "It is more dangerous to be a soldier in the peaceful United States than to have been on the firing-line in France. Is there a military or other emergency that would justify so great a sacrifice of life?" The numbers were truly staggering. At U.S. army camps, one in every four soldiers was sick. On the day Crowder canceled the October draft, 6,139 more soldiers fell ill. In Hoboken, New Jersey, and other ports of embarkation for Europe, deaths from influenza-related pneumonia had reached a stunning 20 percent.

At 9:40 P.M. on Tuesday, October 8, a grim Woodrow Wilson paid a surprise visit upon Army Chief of Staff, General Payton March.

The brash, outspoken General faced his Commander-in-Chief across an oak desk. Elegantly dressed, as always, in a light grey suit, with a pearl stickpin and rimless spectacles, the President said he had received recommendations, "by men whose ability and patriotism are unquestioned," to halt shipments of men to France until the influenza epidemic could be contained. Wilson's concern was genuine. Most Washingtonians, including March, knew that the sedate, professorial President—the former president of Princeton University—read each night from a khaki-bound YMCA Bible given him by an army private. Still, March made his case. Every man embarking for Europe was checked thoroughly for flu. Everything possible was being done to control the spread of the disease. "Despite all this," March conceded, soldiers continued to get sick. "But," he affirmed, "every such soldier who has died [on board ship] has just as surely played his part as his comrade who has died in France." March continued: "In the face of the German Chancellor's appeal, think of the effect on a weakening enemy if they learned that American divisions and replacements were no longer reaching Pershing." Every American who could bear arms must be shipped to Europe "as a show of strength." "The shipment of troops should not be stopped for any cause," the General concluded emphatically.

Years later, Payton March remembered: "President Wilson turned in his chair and gazed out the window. The sacrifice of the lives of all these fine Americans distressed him to the soul. He gave a faint sigh and nodded. Then his eyes twinkled and he said, 'General, I wonder if you have heard this limerick: 'I had a little bird and its name was Enza...'"

Wilson made his decision. Shipments of troops to Europe would continue. March cabled Pershing: "If we are not stopped on account of influenza, which has passed the 200,000 mark, you will get replacements by 30 November."

In Washington, D.C., the crisis deepened. The city's "Health Czar," Dr. H.S. Mustard, pleaded for volunteers, "Helpers and more helpers." Quoting from Buddha, he chastised those who would not help: "All men serve their stricken brother save those who deserve not the name of man!" Then Mustard fell sick with influenza. So did his friend and ally, City Commissioner Louis Brownlow.

In his family's funeral home, six-year-old Bill Sardo was asked to "serve" just like everyone else. The house had become a maze of coffins and bodies. Only Bill's father (and sometimes not even he) remembered who was lying where.

> When grieving relatives came to see their loved one, my father would tell me, "Go up to the second floor, and in the third row of the living room or the fourth row of the dining room you'll find a body. Take these people there." So I would lead them through the house, past all the other bodies, to where their beloved was resting.

Late one evening, in another part of the nation's capital, U.S. Congressman Jacob Meeker, forty years old, stood beside his long-time secretary. The two were wed in a small private ceremony. Bride, groom, judge, and witnesses all wore masks. Congressman Meeker died of influenza seven hours later.

In his aunt and uncle's house in Lincoln, Illinois, William Maxwell slept and slept. He remembers:

> Time was a blur. I was sleeping in my uncle's study and I would wake up and it would be daylight and then I would wake up

and it would be dark. I had no sense of day and night. I had a high fever. I felt sick and hollow inside. My mother was in the hospital in Bloomington. The baby had been born. I knew my mother had Spanish influenza and double pneumonia. What I didn't know was that my father had Spanish influenza as well and was very sick. I knew what was going on because my room was near the head of the stairs and I could hear the telephone. One day I overheard my aunt say the dreadful phrase, "She's doing as well as can be expected." I've never heard that used except in circumstances where the worst was about to happen.

On the third day after the baby was born, my mother died. My father called my aunt and asked her to tell us. I heard the telephone conversation from my room. I heard her say, "Will, oh, no," and then, "If you want me to." She came into my room and took me into my grandmother's room. I sat on my grandmother's lap. My aunt brought my brother into the room. She tried to tell us what had happened, but tears ran down her face, so she didn't need to tell me. I knew that the worst that could happen had happened. My mother was marvelous and when she died the shine went out of everything.

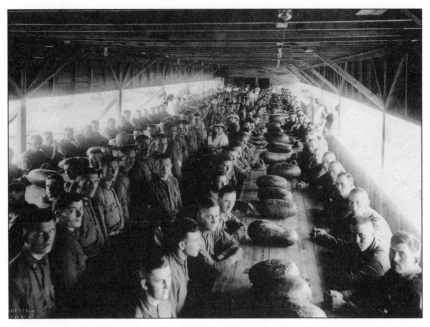

In 1918, with America at war, the epidemic exploded through crowded troop camps.

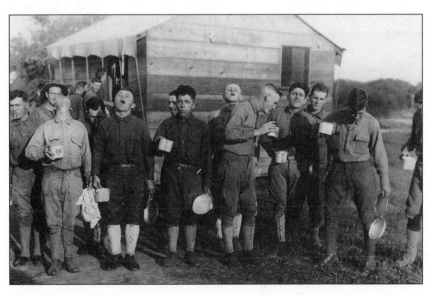

Recruits gargled with salt water to ward off the mysterious disease.

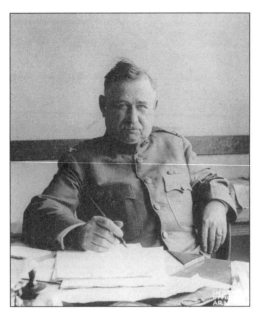

U.S. Surgeon General Rupert Blue, a grizzled veteran of the war against yellow fever and bubonic plague, had never seen anything like this. Boston was struck first; flu quickly engulfed the nation. Local authorities pleaded for federal help, but Blue's Public Health Service possessed only a handful of doctors and researchers, and no funds for epidemic control.

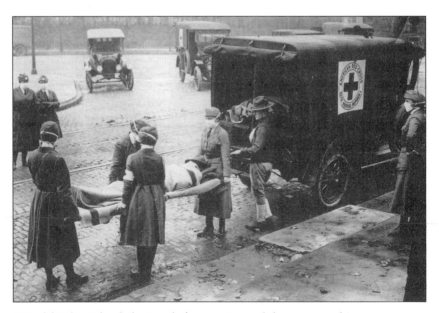

World War I had drained the nation of doctors and nurses. The American Red Cross and scores of other private organizations pitched in.

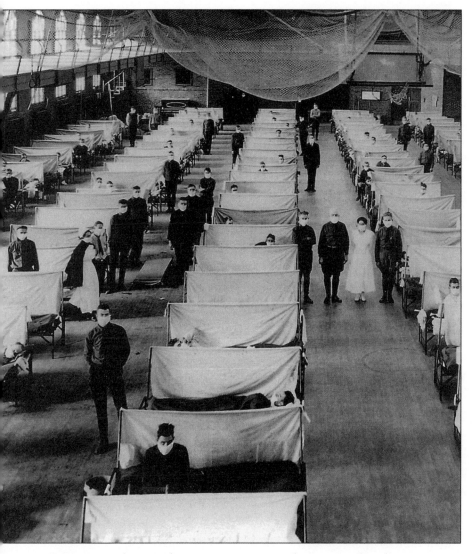

Emergency hospitals sprang up everywhere, in schools,
churches, auditoriums, even dance halls and county jails.
Sheets strung between cots in a gymnasium represent a crude
attempt to isolate highly-infectious patients.

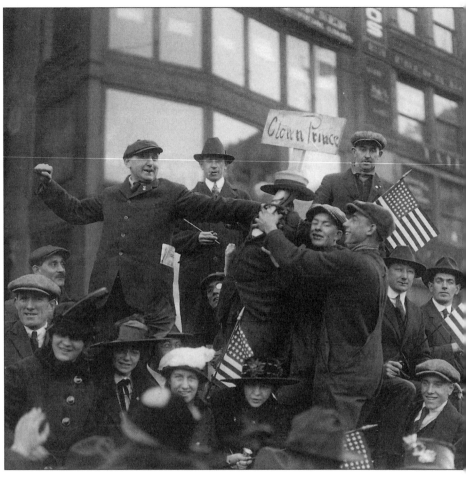

Despite the epidemic, war fever continued to burn. Many
Americans blamed the Germans for the scourge, believing
U-boats had released the "germs" on America's shores. Here,
patriots display an effigy of Prince Max of Baden, Germany's
Imperial Chancellor.

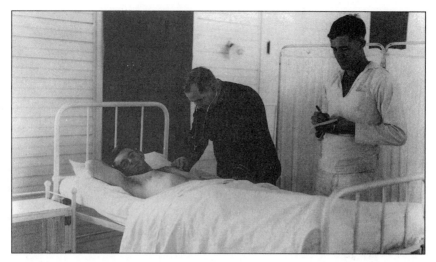

Medical men were bewildered by the disease. Spanish influenza often felled its victims in a matter of hours, causing every organ in the body to fail. Lungs filled with bloody fluid, and patients asphyxiated.

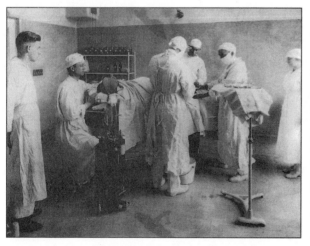

By today's standards, medicine in 1918 was a crude science. Although most doctors acknowledged they were helpless against the disease, argument raged over treatment. "Cures" included whiskey, cigars, milk toast, and nebulous, intriguing concoctions like "Grippura." Some physicians doused their patients with icy water. Others resorted to the ancient practice of "bleeding" patients. Still others tried surgery, slicing open a patient's chest, spreading his ribs, and extracting a quotient of pus and blood.

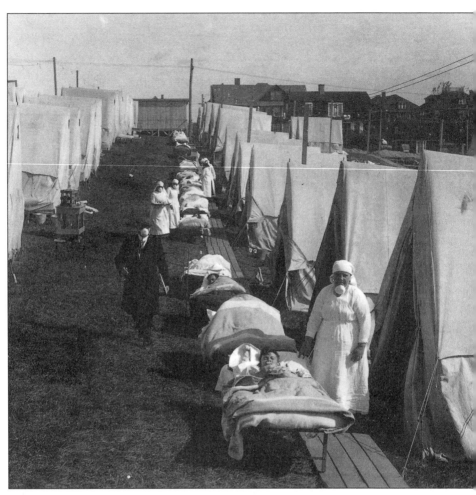

Tents pitched in a grassy field house the overflow from packed hospitals. Advocates of a "fresh air" cure became increasingly vocal. Indeed, the death rate among patients on Boston's breezy Corey Hill was significantly lower than the stunning 50-percent mortality reported in area hospitals.

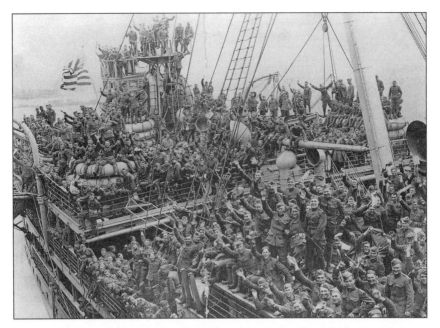

Crammed troopships played perfect host to a breath-borne disease. Many troopships became floating "death-houses." Despite this, President Woodrow Wilson decided on October 8, 1918, to keep troops moving to Europe.

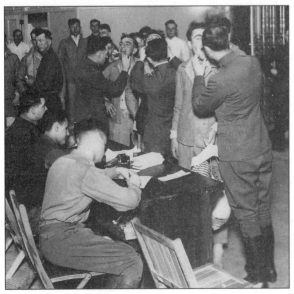

Weary doughboys arriving in France are checked for traces of flu.

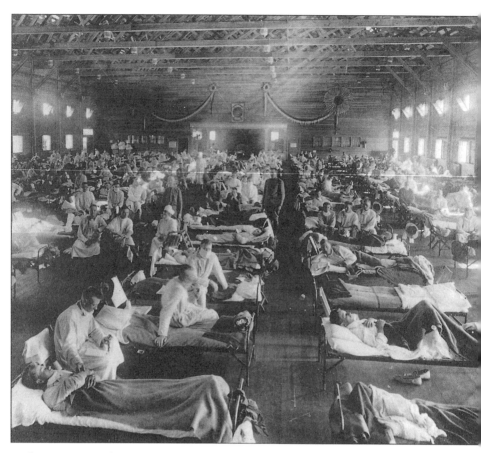

Influenza sent the mortality rate in the U.S. Army soaring.

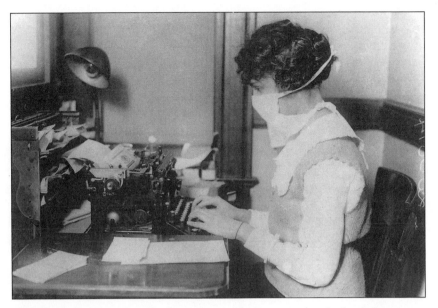

In America, face masks became a ubiquitous symbol of the invisible threat.

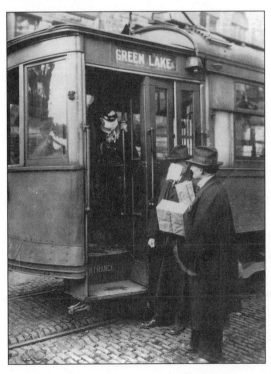

A "mask-slacker" is turned away from a trolley.

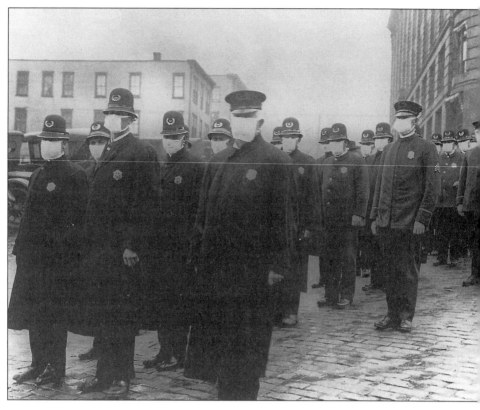

As cities shut down, policemen, firemen, schoolteachers, and city employees manned soup kitchens, hospitals, morgues, and graveyards. In Seattle, masked policemen warily await orders.

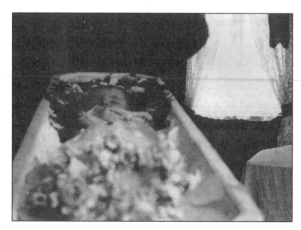

Immigrants in crowded, urban ghettos were especially vulnerable to the disease. An immigrant baby is laid out at home, in Lawrence, Massachusetts.

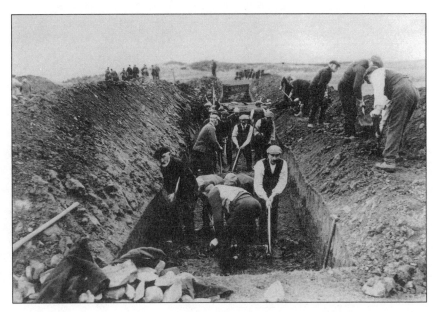

Gravediggers struggle to hew a trench from a rocky field.

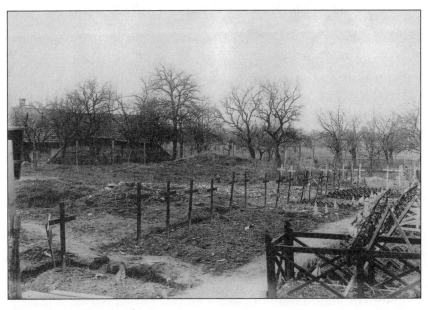

A grave site in Utah.

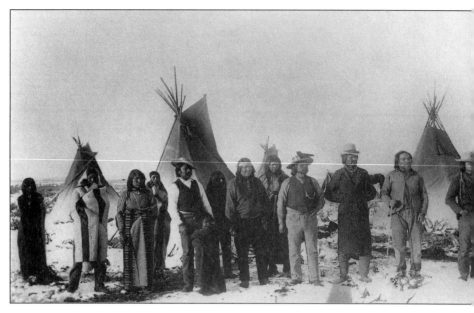

Ute Indians, Utah. Native Americans died at a rate four times the national average.

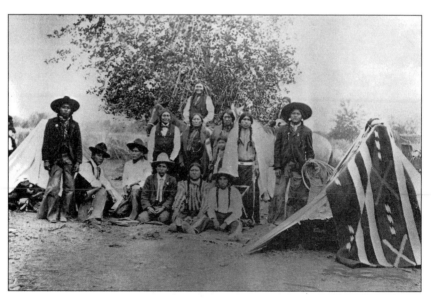

Ute Indian life, like that of Alaska's Eskimos, revolved around rituals of communality and sharing. Flu decimated Ute camps.

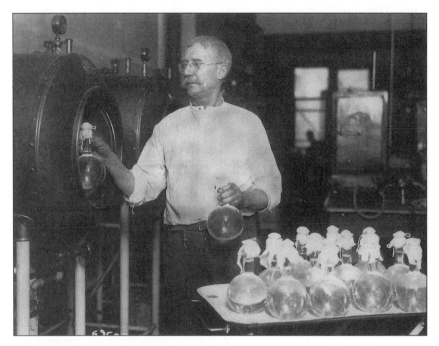

Scientists, believing Spanish influenza was caused by a bacteria, feverishly concocted vaccines.

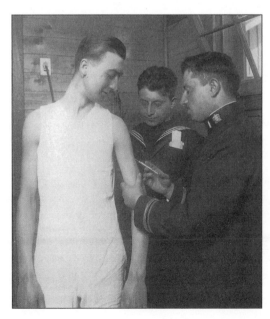

Dozens of different vaccines were shot into hundreds of thousands of arms. Because influenza is caused by a virus, not a bacteria, these vaccines were utterly useless.

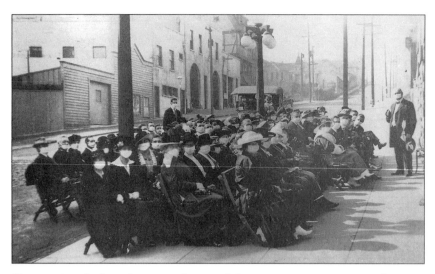

Determined church-goers, banned from congregating inside, hold a sidewalk service in San Francisco.

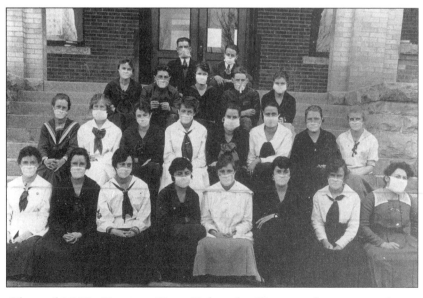

Class of 1918, Canton City, Colorado. Despite the scores of dead, many people adapted quickly to this strange new world.

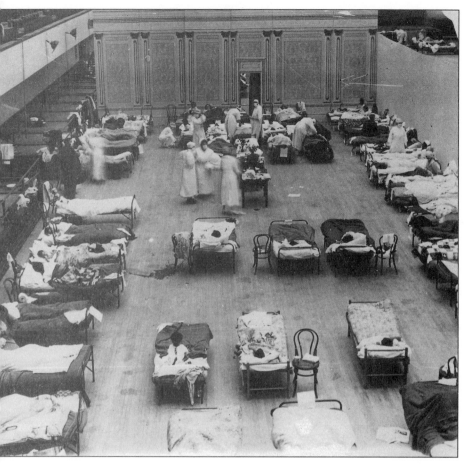

Women bed down in a civic auditorium in Oakland, California.

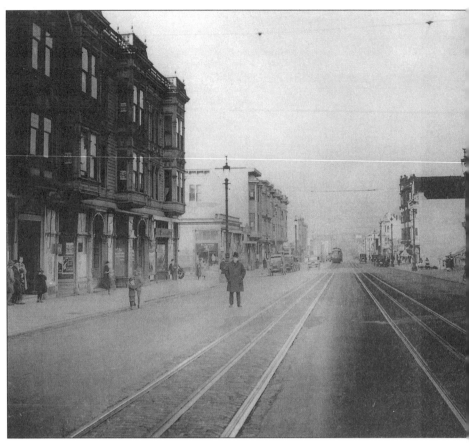

In some places, the epidemic ended swiftly, just as the Armistice stilled the guns in Europe. In other places, like San Francisco, the epidemic died out slowly, erratically. Here, a masked man waits for a trolley on Valencia Street in San Francisco.

Chapter 5

Engagement

An increasingly grim group of medical researchers confronted the global pandemic. Public health officials, physicians, and the American public turned to the triumphant priests of twentieth-century medicine with dazed confusion and a rising sense of panic and betrayal. Science had enjoyed a meteoric rise. The brave new world of medicine had wrought genuine miracles: vaccines, pasteurization, and an understanding of pathologic processes and how disease was spread. Modern science had dispelled mysteries which had bedeviled mankind for millenniums. The fluorescent flash of Roentgen's x-rays, the sophisticated devices of modern surgery, and the powerful lenses of optical microscopes were causing the subtle and ingenious anatomies of the human body to relinquish their stubborn secrets. To many, science represented a new, "modern" version of God. How, if science was all it claimed to be, could a "homey," familiar little illness bring medicine and the modern world to its knees? Earth was engulfed in an epidemic eerily reminiscent of the long-distant past. Had science no more to offer than the crude medical practitioners of medieval Europe? The plague seemed even more incredible when one considered the context. Most scientists believed they knew the cause of influenza. The microbial culprit had been "apprehended" a quarter-century ago: Pfeiffer's bacillus, a rod-shaped bacterium, one-sixteenth the size of a red corpuscle. Why, then, were vaccines, the "magic bullets" of microbiology, failing? Many were being tried. In Illinois alone, eighteen different vaccines were being used. In San Francisco, over eighteen thousand people were inoculated. But in every case, the magic bullets of modern science were missing their mark.

A vaccine is a dose of an infectious agent which provokes a mild, harmless episode of disease, thereby rendering a person immune to that disease. An effective vaccine depends upon the precise identification of the causative agent. In the fall of 1918, in laboratories all over the world, medical researchers feverishly concocted vaccines which contained a host of bacterial agents: staphylococcus, streptococcus, pneumococcus, and many others. In this game of pure guesswork, only one variable remained constant. Invariably, the vaccines featured Pfeiffer's bacillus.

But if Pfeiffer's bacteria was truly the cause of Spanish influenza, why were vaccines proving useless? Had Pfeiffer simply gotten it wrong?

Britain's illustrious Dr. John Eyre sternly reprimanded his colleagues for their doubt. Eyre wrote:

> The epidemic is one of true influenza, due to *bacillus influenzae* [Pfeiffer's bacillus], complicated in a large percentage of cases by secondary infections with pneumococcus or streptococcus longus. I fail to understand the attitude of those who, confronted with the available data, refuse to accept the obvious and seek some mysterious and elusive pathological virus, filter-passer, or what not, to explain a pandemic which is the exact counterpart of the one which a quarter of a century ago prompted the investigation which led to the discovery of *bacillus influenzae*.

Other scientists sounded wary echoes of the past.

> I have arrived at the conclusion that if our scientists were to make a careful chemical, geological, and meteorological survey

of the countries now affected by the so-called influenza, some irritated condition of the atmosphere would be found which would account for the cause and rapid extension of this ailment. Influenza is in reality a non-bacterial, non-contagious disease caused by the inhalation of small amounts of a depressing, highly irritating, high density gas, present in the atmosphere, especially at night and when the air is surcharged with moisture.

—Dr. Albert J. Croft, Chicago

In the laboratories of New York's Rockefeller Institute, Dr. Martha Wollstein set to work. Like other medical researchers, Wollstein resolved to identify the microbe responsible for Spanish influenza. But her methodical research only led her deeper into the heart of a riddle. Reports from all over the world seemed to contradict Pfeiffer's findings. A potpourri of bacteria were being recovered from influenza victims, often in far greater amounts than Pfeiffer's bacillus. In some cases, Pfeiffer's bacteria was nowhere to be found, a finding which puzzled even Pfeiffer himself. Wollstein determined that "Pfeiffer's bacillus is a frequent invader of the human body, where it either causes or complicates important pathological processes." Pfeiffer's bacillus was also common in animals (especially rabbits), but its pathologic threat differed widely, depending upon the animal host. Still, was Pfeiffer's bacillus alone enough to explain the bewildering savagery of Spanish influenza? Was Spanish influenza even *influenza* at all?

The disease was downright bizarre. No organ in the human body was spared. When had influenza produced complete, catastrophic bodily failure, such swift demise and death? When had influenza caused inflammation of the entire body, with air or gas collecting beneath the skin? When had the flu caused coma, spastic twitching of muscles and tendons, paralysis of the eye muscles or otitis media (where the middle ear cavity becomes choked with pus)? Coughs which produced pints of yellow-green pus were sometimes so violent they tore the muscles of the rectum. Urinary retention resulted in the puffy faces and swollen ankles of acute nephritis. Urine output was reduced to a dribble of smoky, blood-streaked liquid. Through a stethoscope, lungs sounded (according to one doctor) "like a bank note being crisped in a pocket." Autopsies were revealing truly horrific findings, what one physician called "a pathological nightmare." Swollen hearts, riddled with fat, weighed 13 ounces, 4 ounces above normal. Lungs were riddled with nodules "as big as hens' eggs." Lungs weighed up to six times normal and looked "like melted red currant jelly."

On a brisk October afternoon, Dr. Joseph Goldberger, a lanky, resolute U.S. Public Health Service researcher, addressed a group of convicts at a naval prison in Massachusetts. Goldberger was seeking volunteers for a "special program": "certain influenza experiments." If the prisoners completed the program, they would be pardoned of their crimes. Out of a thousand convicts, sixty-eight volunteered—an astonishing number, given the fact that Goldberger was about to inject them with Spanish influenza.

Goldberger's goal was simple. He set out to confirm that Pfeiffer's bacillus caused Spanish influenza. Unlike researchers agonizingly searching the pea soup of bacteria culled from the sick or the dead, Goldberger would prove the microbe's guilt by inducing disease in the well.

Thirty-nine brave, desperate volunteers (who, by history, had never had the flu) were chosen as human guinea pigs. The convicts were quarantined on Gallups Island in Boston Harbor. Each man inhaled a pure culture of Pfeiffer's bacillus. Each was then inoculated with blood from flu patients, then with colonies of Pfeiffer's bacillus taken from the lungs of the dead. Nothing happened. No volunteer got sick. Goldberger sprayed the convicts' nostrils and eyes, then swabbed their throats with broths of pure Pfeiffer's bacillus. Again: nothing. New England and

Boston were wracked with flu, but Goldberger's volunteers remained defiantly, impossibly healthy.

Shaken, Goldberger transferred ten of the volunteers to the influenza wards of Chelsea Naval Hospital. Each convict shook hands with ten flu victims, talked with ten flu victims, sat by their bedsides. Finally, the convicts leaned up close and let dying patients cough in their faces. Again, no volunteers got sick.

Shockingly, not one of the thirty-nine volunteers got the flu. But Goldberger's colleague, the doctor who ran the quarantine station, caught influenza and died.

A similar test was undertaken in San Francisco. For one month, fifty sailors were quarantined in a Naval Training Station on Yerba Buena Island in San Francisco Bay. They were then moved to an even more remote location, Angel Island, also in San Francisco Bay. For one month, Angel Island's fifty sailors suffered a barrage of bacilli. Pfeiffer's bacillus and many others were injected and infused in a myriad of ways. Three of the volunteers developed tonsillitis. Again, in defiance of all logic, not one of the sailors came down with flu.

The irony was painful. Public Health Service scientists were unable to give influenza to willing, compliant volunteers, even as Americans were dying by the hundreds of thousands.

A highly contagious, infectious disease, influenza is spread primarily through coughs and sneezes. In a single sneeze, eighty-five million bacteria and forty-six hundred viral particles explode into the air. Hurling at a "muzzle velocity" of 152 feet per second, up to a distance of 12 feet, they linger in the air for more than half an hour. One air-borne, mucousy droplet can spawn nineteen thousand colonies of bacteria. Hurtling alongside these bacterial "giants" are the minuscule viral agents of influenza. Twelve million influenza viruses can fit on the head of a pin.

We know today that microbes enter the human body through the nasal passages on tiny airborne droplets, expelled in coughs and sneezes. We know today that influenza is caused by a virus, not a bacteria—neither Pfeiffer's nor anyone else's. Still, the experiments in Boston and San Francisco *should* have produced influenza. Why didn't they? Perhaps each volunteer had unwittingly suffered a mild case of flu the previous spring and had acquired immunity. Influenza viruses are infinitely delicate; a day or two following infection, the fragile strands of RNA (ribonucleic acid) which compose a virus are shed from the body. Perhaps the nasal and respiratory secretions culled from victims and given to volunteers no longer contained active influenza virus. Still, that not one of the eighty-seven human guinea pigs got sick testifies to the near-impossibility of using human beings as scientific "laboratory animals."

In mid-October, Dr. Martha Wollstein published the results of her exhaustive research. "The patients' reactions," she reported, "are not sufficiently clear-cut to signify that Pfeiffer's bacillus is the specific inciting agent." In other words, her findings were inconclusive. Teams of researchers at St. Mary's Hospital in London and the New York City Department of Health made a similarly discouraging announcement: "Our final conclusion is, therefore, that the micro-organism causing the epidemic has not yet been identified." On October 5, 1918, the prestigious *Journal of the American Medical Association* declared, "The 'influence' in influenza is still veiled in mystery." In November 1918, the *Illinois Health News*, in a dash of black humor, wrote:

> ?Flu?
> If we but knew
> The cause of flu
> And whence it comes and what to do,
> I think that you

And we folks, too,
Would hardly get in such a stew.
Do you?

Medical researchers found themselves bedeviled. To some, it seemed increasingly evident that a minuscule "filterable agent" was at work. In fact, influenza researchers like Martha Wollstein were slowly, arduously, and sometimes inadvertently inventing the science of virology. In odd, ingenious, and often bewilderingly confused experiments in Japan, Germany, France, Great Britain, and the United States, scientists were searching for *something*— they just didn't know what. The word virus is derived from the Latin word for "poison." In 1918, the idea of viruses as we understand them today had not yet been formulated. Some microbiologists used the word to describe toxins (chemicals) produced by bacteria which caused disease, as in diphtheria. Others used the word to describe so-called "filterable agents," the yet-unseen, yet-unproved microbes which were far smaller than bacteria and which could *theoretically* cause disease. Scientists had successfully passed solutions through filters which should have blocked the passage of bacteria. These "filtrates" had then been shown to be infectious. In 1898, this was demonstrated with a plant virus, the tobacco mosaic virus. But in 1918, no experiment had yet revealed the presence of filterable agents in any human disease process.

> In 1918, scientists were looking for a needle in a haystack, only they didn't know it was a needle they were looking for and the needle was too small for them to see anyway. No wonder they didn't find it.
>
> —Alfred Crosby, Historian

The brave new world of medicine had failed. The mystique surrounding the disease deepened.

Urgent pleas for help poured into the United States Public Health Service: "More doctors...more nurses, more face masks...more medicine...more blankets and pneumonia jackets!" Theoretically, the Public Health Service had been created for exactly this sort of crisis; in reality, the crisis was overwhelming. Still, the federal government had taken the offensive. Congress' million-dollar appropriation gave Surgeon General Rupert Blue the money and authority to hire 1,085 doctors and 703 nurses. But no one in this combatant nation had told him where to find them. Blue sent out a call for volunteers to old folks' homes and institutions for the partially disabled. Bit by bit, he filled his quota. One doctor was eighty-five years old. Another had a wooden leg. Another had a drug-addiction problem.

But they would serve. And serve they did. By late October, the Public Health Service had over six hundred doctors fighting the epidemic, most of them literally on the run. One doctor in San Jose, California, did not bother getting in and out of his car; a friend drove while he rode the running board. He saw 525 patients in a single day. In Bennington, Nebraska, Dr. Charles Hickey only took time to sleep in the front seat of his buggy as his faithful horse guided him to the next call. A patient in Enid, Oklahoma, forever remembered a famished Dr. David Harris taking his pulse with one hand, chewing on a snatched drumstick with the other and dribbling broth across the sickbed.

It was the same all over the world. Some villages in Hungary had not seen a doctor for over five years. In England, the doctor to patient ratio was one to five thousand. In France, where all physicians under the age of sixty-five had been drafted into the military, octogenarians dusted off their black bags and gamely set off. In Milan, Italy, Dr. Lorenzini, a frail but intrepid eighty-year-old General Practitioner, was carried piggyback on his rounds by a brawny washer-woman, Ida Carlini. In the town of Oosterbeek in the Netherlands, a consult with the courteous Dr. Gerrit Broekma now involved a shrill shout from the street, "Have any of you got the flu?" followed by the directive, "Don't go into trams, don't visit anyone, don't receive people. If you feel weak, take a strong drink." In Quebec, at least ten thousand patients could not beg, borrow, or steal a physician. In Otterville, Ontario, the situation was somewhat better—farmers were bribing scarce medical men with deeds of land. Anyone who could read a thermometer was drafted into service. In New Orleans, 175 dentists became physicians overnight. Students at the American School of Osteopathy in Kirksville, Missouri, graduated early. In Sacramento, California, ninety-seven candidates were approved by the State Board of Medical Examiners in a single day. In Reykjavik, Iceland, veterinarians made a speedy transition from doctoring sheep to treating humans. Egyptians were reviving the rather ominous medieval tradition of the "barber surgeon."

The European War had drained the world of doctors. Given the twin catastrophes of war and influenza, doctors were as rare in France as hen's teeth. In Amiens, France, Lieutenant Ivo Cobb welcomed a "real doctor" to the Royal Army Medical Corps only to discover that the retired Major had forgotten which end of a stethoscope to hold against a patient's chest. In Dorset, England, Flight-Lieutenant Halliday Sutherland, ordered to inspect two thousand airmen in two hours for traces of influenza, sped through the ranks, randomly checking pulse rates, then collapsed in the mud, stricken with flu. Influenza was everywhere. A convoy of eight vessels limped into St. Nazaire, France, with a cargo of 2,873 sick; 265 had been buried at sea. A.E.F. hospitals in Europe were "107 percent full," crammed with patients tagged "three-day fever." Influenza had sent the mortality rate in the U.S. Army soaring from 4.4 to 89.9 deaths per thousand. The *Baltimore Sun* reported:

Spanish influenza is playing havoc with the Army, notwith-
standing all the precautions to prevent its spread and the ap-
plication of the best medical science to it. Last week, 88,478
new cases of the disease were reported, as against 37,845 for
the preceding week. There were more than 8,000 additional
cases of pneumonia. This is an increase of 100 percent.

Doctors, nurses, hospital beds, and ambulances were all scarce.
Medical attention was not only rare; often, it was a mixed blessing. Hospitals were useful to the well because they functioned as
quarantines. Many, however, were little better than death
houses. The poor were often dragged into hospitals by force, not
for cure or mercy, but to isolate the violently-ill from society. For
those in hospitals, there were no guarantees. In Boston, the hospital death rate rose to a stunning all-time high of 50 percent.
Across the Atlantic, in immaculate Zurich, Switzerland, one-
third of all hospital patients developed pneumonia. In Denmark,
Dr. Victor Scheel of Bispebjerg Hospital urged the sick to stay
home. "It is best not to move the patient to hospital. The contagion is so strong that official measures are purely illusory."

Even when they could only provide an "illusion" of knowledge, physicians, like medical researchers, played their hunches.
Major Walter Brem of the U.S. Army Medical Corps claimed
morphine reduced respiration rate. Others argued morphine
dried up the lungs' natural secretions. In Greece and Austria,
physicians injected patients with mercury perchloride; others
warned this could damage gastric function. Some doctors championed quinine and strychnine; others claimed strychnine increased a patient's delirium. In Alexandria, Virginia, the town's
two remaining doctors visited hundreds of patients a day, dis-
pensing their own brand of "flu cure": atropine capsules (a distil-
late of belladonna) and whiskey. Physicians in India and England
dispensed vast quantities of aspirin, the new "miracle drug." But

did aspirin weaken hearts, leaving a patient vulnerable to pneumonia? Some patients were given a syrup of sodium benzoate and crushed foxglove or an expectorant made of pine resin. Dr. Louis Dechmann of Seattle suggested soaking towels in hot vinegar and placing them on the abdomen: "The acetic acids of vinegar is absorbed through the pores and transformed into acetate, which will prevent coagulation of the blood." One's diet should consist of egg punch, custard, graham crackers, and milk toast. Dr. A. Crichton of Castleton, Ontario, concocted a brew called "Grippura." It cured flu as well as rheumatism, typhoid fever, whooping cough, and scarlet fever. One Midwestern General Practitioner passed out pills in three pretty colors. They were sugar pills—placebos. Why? He felt he had to do *something*. Of the pharmaceutical free-for-all, Chicago's Dr. James B. Herrick warned bitterly, "This is poly-pharmacy run riot."

Still, desperate doctors and desperate patients played on. In Richmond, Virginia, Dr. Bernard Reams soaked the legs and feet of flu victims in tubs of scalding water, then swaddled his patients in blankets until they were beet-red. In Sweden, Dr. Karl Gronstedt preferred icy sheets, camphor injections, and soap-and-water enemas. Like his colleague to the north, Dr. Roland "Kill or Cure" Burkitt believed in the "cold sheet" theory. His patients in Nairobi were confined to freezing beds and doused in icy water.

In England, factory doctors swore tobacco was a "germicide." Smoking became permitted in war-plants. Pro-tobacco Australian pathologists performed autopsies in a blue haze of pipe-smoke. In Zwolle, Holland, grocer Johan Zijlstra ordered his staff to smoke cigars as his doctor had advised. Every one of Zijlstra's employees became sick, except one who had refused to smoke on religious grounds. While tobacco seemed to many a reasonable prophylactic, liquor was hotly debated. The British Royal College of Physicians declared sternly, "Alcohol invites disaster." The Danes banned liquor, except by prescription. But all over the world, patients wanted a drink, and for many physicians, whiskey was one of the few "tricks" left in their little black bags. In the United States, the price of whiskey soared. In Canada, hundreds waited in line for alcohol "upon prescription." In Danzig, Poland, medicinal brandy inebriated the sick and healthy alike. In Wellington, New Zealand, the Mayor himself, His Worship J.P. Luke, dispensed the city's stash of liquor from the parlor of his home.

A cure? Wishful thinking. In central Arkansas, a doctor told a patient's wife, "This is my twenty-fifth case. I've lost the first twenty-four." Some doctors lost their bedside manner entirely. A twelve-year-old in Pueblo, Colorado forever remembered his doctor's bitter advice, "Get on the waiting list for a casket."

Doctors simply did not know what to do. Some welcomed the inky blood gushing from the noses of flu victims, believing it represented a cathartic "venting of poisoned blood." Others turned to thoracic surgery. Making an incision in the chest cavity (where pus was collecting around the ribs), surgeons would remove a section of rib and insert a drainage tube. Recovering patients were forced to blow feebly on children's trumpets to expel the residual fluid. Other doctors resorted to venesection, the ancient practice of bleeding patients. Surgeon General Rupert Blue issued a warning: "The Health Service urges the public to remember that remedies now being recommended do more harm than good." But there was nothing Blue himself could recommend. He conceded, "There is as yet no specific cure for influenza."

Like Rupert Blue, seven-year-old Dan Tonkel of Goldsboro, North Carolina, had a keen grasp of the obvious.

> The medical world did not know how to handle the disease. Doctors didn't have any medicines or vaccines. And since doctors didn't have the cure-all in their little black satchel, there was very little they could do.
>
> —Dan Tonkel

We didn't know of any medications. There were no such things as pills or medicine. There were no doctors. A traveling nurse went around to houses in my neighborhood, but she didn't know much about the disease either.

—John Deleno of New Haven, Connecticut

Where medicine failed, perhaps hope and prayer would work— or superstition. In the fall of 1918, folk cures flourished and proliferated. "Cures" were concocted of red peppers, of chloroform, asparagus, kerosene, strychnine. Onions proved a popular panacea. A woman in Cleveland advised: "Cut up two large onions and add to them rye flour, make it into a cake, wrap it in a thin white cloth and apply it to the chest.... That night I was so fine. The next day the influenza was gone." Another woman dosed her desperately-sick daughter with onion syrup, then encased her from head to toe in an eye-watering bed of raw onions. The girl survived. A woman in South Chicago suggested peppers. "Take two or three large, ripe red peppers, chop fine, set on the stove and boil nicely for an hour or more. The vapor kills the germs of disease." She conceded that "In some cases, a second treatment might be needed." A man in Halifax, Nova Scotia, suggested drinking fourteen gins in quick succession. Others championed poultices of goose grease and a bag of asafoetida worn around the neck.

A rank, bitter, resinous material derived from the roots of plants of the genus *Ferula*, asafoetida was a popular folk preventative in 1918. In North Carolina, Dan Tonkel endured a bag of asafoetida around his neck: "It smelled to high heaven. People thought the smell would kill germs. So we all wore a bag of asafoetida and smelled like rotten flesh." In Philadelphia, Harriet Ferrel suffered a similar fate. Harriet's neighbors were concocting all kinds of "cures." She remembers:

We made medicines from herbs, from tree bark. We mixed

the seeds of a plant from North Carolina with sulfur. We made all different kinds of teas. We also tried turpentine on sugar and kerosene on sugar. We hung bags of asafoetida or garlic about our necks. We smelled awful, but it was okay, because everyone smelled bad.

In New Haven, John Deleno still knocked every morning on the door of his friends' houses. He still waited for someone to answer. But no one did. "I didn't know what was happening. Finally, my mother told me God had taken them. My friends had gone to Heaven."

Nurse Josie Mabel Brown had taken the Pullman from St. Louis to her assignment at the Great Lakes Naval Training Center armed only with a basket of chicken and cake. She arrived upon a scene of chaotic horror. She was assigned to a ward of forty-two beds. In each bed, a soldier was dying. Lying on stretchers on the floor, other boys were waiting for the boys in the beds to die.

Given the lack of a pharmaceutical or therapeutic cure, nurses were arguably more valuable than doctors and even more scarce. It was nurses who performed the small tasks which saved lives, providing a sip of water, a warm blanket, warm food. Like many nurses, Josie Mabel Brown worked eighteen-hour days, sometimes more. But selflessness and enthusiasm did not guarantee success. Brown's niece, Carla Morrisey, later recounted the stories her aunt had told her about that dreadful autumn. "We would give them a little hot whiskey toddy," Brown had said. "That's about all we had time to do. We didn't have time to treat them." Brown never forgot the suffering she witnessed. "When their lungs collapsed, air was trapped beneath their skin. As we rolled the dead in winding sheets, their bodies crackled—an awful crackling noise which sounded like Rice Crispies when you pour milk over them." Brown functioned, as she saw it, as an ineffective middleman between ambulance and morgue.

> An ambulance would arrive, carrying four litters. It would bring us four live soldiers, and take away four dead ones. The morgues were packed almost to the ceiling with bodies stacked one on top of another. The morticians worked day and night.

Even when she was trying to sleep, Nurse Brown heard the noise of trucks backing up to the morgue, hauling away the dead.

Like Josie Mabel Brown, nurses everywhere worked to exhaustion. In Canaan, Connecticut, public health nurse Edith L. Price felt "like a machine going about until I ran down." At New York's Columbia Presbyterian Hospital, Nurse Dorothy Deming felt "as truly under fire as though we were with our brothers in the Argonne." The misery continued day and night. Nurse Deming could only sleep if masked with a black silk stocking, her ears plugged with cotton wool.

In the backwoods of Michigan's Upper Peninsula, a public health nurse named Annie Colon and a physician used a handcar to reach isolated cases in remote logging camps. The two pumped the vehicle's hand levers up and down, endlessly riding the rails—armed with whiskey, gin, rum, aspirin, quinine, cough syrup, soup, blankets, even children's toys. "We worked day and night. We'd ride twenty and thirty miles at night through the deepest woods. We would find ten people all huddled together fully dressed in a tiny log cabin, all in two beds and all with fevers over 104 degrees." Often, to save a patient, further improvisation was necessary. "We'd hitch a flat-car to a handcar with wire, put a board floor on, mattresses over that, plenty of covers and a canvas to cover the top and break the wind, and we'd carry patients fifteen or more miles to a decent bed and a chance to live...."

Everybody worked hard and long with unselfish spirit." Doctors and nurses milked cows, made fires, washed and dressed the sick and helpless. In Oregon, as in Michigan, public health nurses struggled to reach victims in remote parts of the state. One nurse reported from the hamlet of Denio:

> Our patients are mostly families of sheep herders; they live in miserable cabins scattered in most inaccessible places, a house to a hill and each hill from twelve to fifteen miles apart. There is no food, no bedding, and absolutely no conception of the first principles of hygiene, sanitation, or nursing care.
>
> I have taken over the hotel as a hospital and the Big Boss, who employs the sheep herders, is having all who are not too ill to be moved in here. The men are willing, some are intelligent, but most are sick. If not for the grit and brains of the nurses who working here and for the women of the community, God help us!
>
> I am working by fits and starts, as I can snatch a minute off to jot down our needs, hoping that the situation may be clear to you and that you will be able to get us some supplies before we get snowed in for the winter. Our greatest need (next to fruit and malted milk) is feeding cups and drinking tubes, also need lots of gauze and cheesecloth and cotton for pneumonia jackets; also gallons of formaldehyde, if we are to stamp out the disease.

Despite their limited arsenal, doctors and nurses were often seen as saviors, as sources of awesome power—the power over life and death. On the Scottish island of Yell, patients seeking medical attention died in the bedroom of the island's only doctor, Dr. Harry Pearson Taylor, as he deliriously battled a fever. Dr. John Hogan, of Baltimore, was about to enter an apartment in Clifton Park when a group of women on the street spied his black doctor's bag. They ran toward Hogan, almost knocking him over, clawing at his jacket, tearing at his sleeves: "Doctor!

Doctor! Do something, give us something, doctor!" Hogan, terrified, ran away, into the dark night.

"Dignified and discerning women stood on the steps at Altman's and Tiffany's Fifth Avenue shops and accosted passers-by." The women passed out handbills, asking for volunteers. All that was needed was "willingness and courage." Hundreds answered the call. So reported Miss Lillian Wald of New York City, whose Henry Street Settlement House had been at the hurricane center of the epidemic since the beginning. Elsewhere in the city, even the elite pitched in. Mrs. William Randolph Hearst and other socialites baked custards and answered calls for help, speeding through the city in their big cars as members of a "flying squad." Eleanor Roosevelt, whose husband, five children, and three servants were all sick with flu or pneumonia, delivered food to Red Cross hospitals. In Chicago, a society woman arrived for volunteer work dressed completely in gold—a gold tinsel dress, gold bonnet, gold muff, gold slippers. She explained it was her "resurrection dress." She wanted to be to be ready for heaven at any moment.

A Red Cross handbill entreated:

A STERN TASK FOR STERN WOMEN

There is nothing in the epidemic of SPANISH
INFLUENZA to inspire panic.

There is everything to inspire coolness and courage and
sacrifice on the part of American women.

A stern task confronts our women—not only trained
women, but untrained women.

The housewife, the dietitian, the nurses' aide, the prac-

tical nurse, the undergraduate nurse and the trained
nurse herself—all of these are needed.

HUMANITY CALLS UPON THEM

LIVES DEPEND UPON THEIR ANSWER

Capable, though untrained hands, can lighten the burden of the trained ones. There are many things intelli-
gent women can do to relieve the situation, working
under the direction of competent nurses.

WILL YOU HELP DO SOME OF THEM?

WILL YOU ENROLL FOR SERVICE NOW?

Nurse Gertrude Williamson of Wilkes-Barre, Pennsylvania answered the call. She was placed in charge of a Red Cross emergency hospital. She reported:

> For two days, volunteers worked like beavers, cutting draw-
> sheets, making up the Army cots, scrubbing hat-racks to serve as
> linen shelves and cleaning camp chairs to be used as bedside ta-
> bles. The Armory was scrubbed from roof to basement and four
> wards were partitioned off with beaverboard, and lavatories and
> sinks were installed in the only available rooms. The Red Cross
> Canteen Service took entire charge of the basement kitchen
> and, with a few paid employees, but mostly volunteers, served
> the nurses, the physicians, the orderlies, and the members of the
> National Guard who were always on duty, besides sending out
> food, broths mostly, to over 150 families daily, who because of
> the flu had no one well enough to prepare their meals.

In Philadelphia, the Automobile Club and private individuals
provided "ambulances." Off-duty policemen carried stretchers. In

San Francisco, idled school teachers served as nurses, telephone operators, and laundry workers. Soup kitchens, ladling out free food, sprang up everywhere. City offices closed, releasing their employees to volunteer service. The sick were bedded down in emergency hospitals in all kinds of buildings: a Masonic Temple in Waterbury, Connecticut; the Civic Auditorium in San Francisco; a county jail in Arizona. In Enderline, Nebraska, a dilapidated railway hotel became the town's hospital, staffed by fifteen teenagers. In another town, patients were removed to a dance hall; the men's bathroom functioned as morgue. In still another town, a mailman welcomed influenza victims into the post office and bundled his patients in mail sacks.

Cooperation between the public and private sectors flourished. The Public Health Service coordinated efforts with private organizations like the Salvation Army, the YMCA, the Knights of Columbus, and others. Federal, state, and local buildings were converted into hospitals, often by volunteers.

Even insurance companies got into the act. New York's Metropolitan Life Insurance Company sent a public health worker, Miss Wild, to the besieged town of Berlin, New Hampshire. Miss Wild reported:

> It is hardly possible for me to describe the conditions in this community. I am the only experienced public health worker here with the exception of the staff. Saturday, I cared for forty patients, from four to nine sick in one family. Everything possible is being done. There are only seven doctors in the city. Doctors from near-about towns come in for a few hours each day. Surrounding towns are all afflicted, but not to such an extent as Berlin. There is only one fifty-bed hospital in the city in charge of Catholic sisters, who have given up their own rooms as a temporary pneumonia ward. The sisters are sleeping in the school house.

All across America, life had been disrupted. What was normal, what was expected, what was routine and reassuring had given way to the unbelievable, the ghastly, the tragically unreal. Community life, family life, married life, the lives and play of children ground to a halt or became distorted and dominated by disease and death. As families and communities mobilized to fight the pandemic, an obvious dilemma loomed. In devastated Brockton, the dying and the dead increasingly included the volunteers who had answered the city's desperate call. Nurses Georgena and Winnifred Flemming of Nova Scotia were buried alongside six other nurses from Brockton Hospital. Just as crucial as caring for the sick was the need to control the proliferation of the disease, to safeguard the well. The pandemic could not be controlled unless people refrained from that most necessary and human of impulses: interaction.

All across the country, cities shut down by decree. Closing orders affected everything from churches to pool and dance halls, libraries, saloons, ice cream parlors, and red-light districts. Conventions were canceled. Meetings of clubs and other private and public organizations were postponed. Funerals were tightly regulated or banned altogether.

In Kansas, the Spanish Lady had come home. On a single day, October 4, 1,270 soldiers fell sick at Fort Riley. During the month of October, Dr. Edward Schreiner's crammed hospital treated 11,654 influenza patients. Scores more, with fevers of less than 103 degrees, were turned away. Six-foot, six-inch Martin "Giant" Reichberger and others deemed strong enough to withstand the disease died on the porch of the camp's hospital, soaked by a drenching rainstorm. Inside the hospital's crowded wards, 957 soldiers died.

Kansas was engulfed in flu. Dr. Samuel J. Crumbine, Secretary of the State Board of Health, was a well-known sanitarian; Crumbine had attracted national attention for a "swat the fly" campaign and a crusade to ban the communal drinking cup from railroad cars. Like Washington, D.C.'s Louis Brownlow, Crumbine did not deny or underestimate the danger. He immediately instituted sweeping statewide closures. Localities, large and small, answered Crumbine's call. As flu claimed its first victim in the hamlet of Winfield, the *Daily Courier* announced: "Beginning with the crow of the cock and the rising of the sun Saturday morning October 12, [Winfield] will join the whole state of Kansas under a closing order which will prohibit public gatherings of all kinds." Eventually, closing orders affected some ten thousand businesses in Kansas. Still, as businesses registered the economic shock of the plague and churches remained closed, the voices of protest grew louder. Were the closures fair? More than the legal limit of shoppers often congregated in stores. Why, then, couldn't people congregate in churches? One pastor insisted: "There is no reason why the teaching of the religion of God should be stopped if the people are allowed to cram and jam in the stores of the city." Protesters organized watchdog groups to enforce quarantine limits and to ensure that trams carried no more than the legally-allowed ten people.

Kansas was not alone in its protests. To many Americans, especially church-goers, closures seemed to possess a kind of inequity and illogic. The *Philadelphia Inquirer* asked: "Since crowds gather in congested eating places and press into elevators and hang to the straps of ill-ventilated street cars, it is a little difficult to understand what is to be gained by shutting up well ventilated churches and theaters. The authorities seem to be going daft. What are they trying to do, scare everybody to death?" In retrospect, mortality statistics seem to bear out the instincts of protesters. In some ways, this highly-contagious disease was profoundly predictable, almost inevitable. Controlling contagion on such a scale through quarantines, closures, or the wearing of face masks was virtually impossible. Widespread closures in Washington, D.C., Philadelphia,

St. Louis, and other large cities did little to contain the flu. In some instances, communities with less stringent ordinances fared better than those with strict closing orders.

In this, as in so many ways, Spanish influenza continued to prove profoundly unpredictable. Some communities were devastated, while other similar or nearby ones were spared, a phenomenon which only intensified feelings of panic and helplessness. Public officials had a limited arsenal; they had to use what modest weapons they had. For many, sanitation became an obsession. Phone booths were padlocked. Drinking fountains were "sanitized" by blow-torch hourly. Telephones were doused in alcohol. Firemen endlessly hosed down city streets. Cashiers in groceries and restaurants were required to dip their fingers in disinfectant after each transaction.

For many officials, the face mask became the weapon of choice against the mysterious plague. An omnipresent sign of the times, masks became a pointed symbol of the invisible threat. Policemen wore them. Transit drivers wore them. Workers wore them in offices and factories. In some cities, people were not allowed to board a bus or trolley without one. Newlyweds in San Francisco told a doctor that they had worn masks, and nothing else, when they made love. In Cedar City, Utah, the "Goddess of Liberty" at a Red Cross fund-raiser wore a mask. In a dash of morbid humor, masks in Rockford, Illinois, sported a skull-and-crossbones. In Chicago, Lieutenant Al Haase returned home from the war to marry his sweetheart. At his wedding, everyone—bride, groom, reverend, and guests—wore masks, as required by local ordinance. Al Haase mused: "We have to wear gas masks and many peculiar devices in France, but civil life in America seems to be getting just as complex."

Gauze or cheese-cloth masks were probably minimally effective when used properly. But a few loose layers of gauze posed no serious restraint to swarming microbes. It was like trying to keep out dust with chicken wire. To some, like Washington D.C.'s Dr. H.S. Mustard, this was obvious. Mustard continued to call masks "an absurdity, a menace when worn by the civilian population, military or naval class." California's Dr. John F. Kyle declared: "Masks are for doctors and nurses in an operating room. They look good to the poor innocent patient and the nurses. Influenza gets you going or coming regardless of vaccines or mask." Although most Americans gamely donned the "protective gauze," some remained defiant. In this land of the free, disobedience was to them a native right.

Belief in the mask wavered, but never died. Dr. William Hassler, chief of San Francisco's Board of Health, who had once declared influenza would not reach his city, now decreed: "Every person appearing on the public streets [or] in any public place... shall wear a mask or covering except when partaking of meals." Mayor Rolph concurred: "Whomever leaves his mask behind, dies." The Red Cross distributed masks at an astounding rate, giving out one hundred thousand in four days. Newspaper ads blared: "WEAR A MASK and save your life! A mask is 99 percent Proof against Influenza." The *San Francisco Chronicle* suggested, "The man who wears no mask will likely become isolated, suspected, and regarded as a slacker. Like a man of means without a Liberty Loan button, he'll be shy of friends." "Mask slackers" risked a hefty $100 fine or ten days in jail. Remarkably, everyone wore them, creating a bizarre spectacle. Trials were held outdoors with everyone sporting masks. The mounted police wore masks. Cable cars were full of masked men. San Francisco soon resembled a low-budget sci-fi film.

Hassler himself sported an especially elaborate face mask. The *San Francisco Chronicle* offered a wry assessment of Hassler's mask: "The snout extends partially, like the helmets affected by the French knights at the period of Agincourt, but it is not so protrusive as the metal muzzles. Furthermore, it is sheathed outside in gauze like the common or garden mask more usually adopted by the public." Indeed, the stylish, cosmopolitan city was setting the trends in mask-wear. The fashion-wise noted three styles: the "Agincourt" (like Hassler's), the square, no-frills "Ravioli" (preferred by policemen), and the drapey, scarf-like yashmak, worn primarily by young women.

San Francisco was mobilizing with incredible unity. The city's second weapon was vaccination. A doctor at Tufts Medical College in Massachusetts had developed a promising vaccine. Mayor Rolph wired for a huge shipment. A special envoy carried the package on the fleet Twentieth Century Express. The vaccine rode the rails like the rescuing hero of a silent-screen melodrama. Hassler promised, "Influenza here will be under control within a week."

A fortnight later, after a Herculean effort by volunteers, eighteen thousand San Franciscans had been inoculated—with a vaccine which was utterly useless.

Still, neither William Hassler's San Francisco nor Royal Copeland's New York nor Louis Brownlow's Washington saw the worst.

The Spanish Lady reserved her full horror for another place.

Chapter 6

Chaos

Philadelphia, "City of Brotherly Love," welcomed the Spanish Lady with open arms. In the days following the massive Liberty Loan rallies of late September, 1918, influenza struck Philadelphia with vicious fury. No city in America suffered more.

A chill pierced the salty air. Dewy frost lingered on the grass in the morning. Everywhere in Philadelphia, the rituals of autumn had commenced. Sculls sliced through the still, murky waters of the Schuylkill River. Oaks and sycamores exploded with the dazzling colors of autumn: crimson, purple, burnished gold. Eight-year-old Columba Voltz had returned to school. Liberty Loan rallies in Rittenhouse Square, parades, and "patriotic sings" had filled the neighborhood with noisy excitement. Still, more than anything, Columba loved school. And Columba loved school most of all because of the church bells.

> The parish school was just down the street from my house, next to the church. The church bells were magnificent. They rang jubilantly, joyfully, all the time. The bells were beautiful, and they gave me such joy.

Five days after the massive September 28th Liberty Bond rally, seventy thousand feverish Philadelphians jammed area hospitals. Hundreds of thousands more were turned away. Horse-drawn wagons, pushcarts, taxis, and other makeshift ambulances rattled through the streets of the stunned city, carrying their cargo of the sick, the dying, and the dead. Dr. Wilmer Krusen, Director of the Department of Health and Charities, warned the city against "fright or panic." But in the first week of October, 706 Philadelphians died of Spanish influenza.

In the second week of October, 2,635 died.

In the third week of October, 4,597 died.

By October 3, all schools, churches, theaters, and places of amusement in Philadelphia were closed. An emergency telephone switchboard was established at Strawbridge and Clothier department store. For a nurse, doctor, or undertaker call "Filbert 100." Immediately, the switchboard was jammed. Bell Telephone Company doubled, then quadrupled its lines. By October 7, no amount of telephone wire could rescue "Filbert 100"; 850 "hello girls" were sick with flu.

In Rittenhouse Square, Columba Voltz was terrified. Columba lived across the street from a funeral parlor. She stood at the window, watching as coffins collected on the sidewalk.

> The beautiful bells had stopped ringing. All day long, I watched coffins being carried into the church, accompanied by the low, sad, funeral bells: BONG, BONG, BONG. Only a few people were allowed into the church at a time and the services lasted only a few minutes, just long enough to bless the coffin. Then the casket would be carried out and another one would go in. All day long, the funeral bells tolled: BONG, BONG, BONG. Up and down the street, crepes were hanging on the doors of houses. I knew inside every one of those houses, someone was being laid out. I was very scared and depressed. I thought the world was coming to an end.

Crepe ribbons, symbols of mourning, were hanging in Anna Milani's neighborhood, too. Anna and her brothers and sisters still roamed the block, down Ninth Street to St. Nicholas Church. But the sound of children's games, her father's spontaneous arias, the cajoling bellows of fish vendors and pushcart salesmen had been replaced by an eerie silence or the sound of sobs, hacking coughs, and screams. Crepe ribbons were pinned on the doors of houses. A white ribbon indicated that a child or a young person had died. A black ribbon meant a middle aged person had died; a grey ribbon signified the death of an elderly person. Anna recalls:

> We were children. Naturally, we were curious to discover who had died. We went up and down the street, looking at the crepes, seeing who had died next.

The city was in turmoil. The Board of Health was woefully understaffed and Philadelphia City Hall, although capped with a statue of the city's venerable architect, Benjamin Franklin, housed politicians who were more fluent in favoritism than crisis management. Essential services began to fail. Four hundred and eighty-seven Philadelphia policemen were absent from work. Firemen, garbage collectors, and city administrators fell sick. The Bureau of Child Hygiene was jammed with hundreds of children whose parents were ill, dying, or dead, and orphanages, fearing infection, would not accept them. Bureau officials could only plead with the neighbors who had brought them to take the children in. Medical personnel—the rare doctor or nurse, orderlies, and cooks—were overwhelmed. Many medical personnel fell ill. A desperate plea went out for doctors of any age and physical rigor, doctors who recalled even "a little" medicine. A sense of horror and disbelief shrouded the city. Philadelphia was under siege.

The city's only morgue overflowed. Built to handle thirty-six bodies, the morgue was swamped with more than five hundred. Hundreds of bodies wrapped in blood-stained sheets were piled in rooms and hallways. Most were unembalmed and visibly rotting. Even veteran embalmers refused to enter the building. Because of the stench, the back door was left open, allowing horrified passersby to glimpse the grisly chaos.

In the second week of October, city officials began using a steam shovel to dig trenches in Potter's Field for mass graves. Still, the dead sometimes lay in apartments or gutters for days, abandoned.

Life in Philadelphia quickly came to resemble conditions in fourteenth-century Europe, when the Black Plague turned life into a ghoulish struggle. In the city's sprawling immigrant slums, the bedraggled and the half-dead huddled in line for soup or a crust of bread. People either fled at the sight of visiting nurses, frightened by their white gowns and gauzy masks, or assailed them with desperate pleas for help. One nurse on her rounds found a man dead. His wife lay beside him, with their newborn twins, just a day old. The man had died the day the twins were born.

Even the roaming death carts from the days of the Black Death were reproduced in Philadelphia. Families were ordered to leave their dead on sidewalks, to be picked up and taken to mass graves. After 528 Philadelphians died in a single day, Father Joseph Corrigan, director of the city's Catholic Charities, organized a melancholy convoy of six horse-drawn wagons. Night and day, they combed alleys and back streets for the abandoned dead. Parish volunteers and theology students manned the grim march, carrying shovels and spades, lighting the way with kerosene lanterns. A knock on the door often remained unanswered. Forcing their way inside, Father Corrigan's men would find only dead.

In Harriet Ferrel's neighborhood of poor blacks, death visited nearly every house. Solemn, corpse-filled carts passed through her neighborhood.

People were in a panic. Suffering. Crying. The Board of Health had issued a proclamation that anyone who died had to be left out for the wagons. But it was just too much to bear—having to put your loved one on the street for a truck to take them away.

In a poor Jewish enclave in North Philadelphia, Selma Epp's entire family fell sick. She remembers:

My parents went for help. They stood in line for hours outside Pennsylvania Hospital, but were turned away. So they came home and made up their own remedies, like castor oil, laxatives. My grandfather made wine. Nothing helped. Everyone in my family—my parents, grandparents, my aunts, and my brother Daniel—everyone up and down our block was sick. There were no medicines, no doctors, nothing people could do to heal themselves. My grandfather was very religious. He was an Orthodox Jew and he wore his tallith shawl and he prayed, hoping God would take away the illness. Everyone in our house grew weaker and weaker. Then my brother Daniel died. My aunt saw the horse-drawn wagon coming down the street. The strongest person in our family carried Daniel's body to the sidewalk. Everyone was too weak to protest. There were no coffins in the wagon, just bodies piled on top of each other. Daniel was two; he was just a little boy. They put his body in the wagon and took him away.

On October 16, 711 Philadelphians died of Spanish influenza. More people died on that day than on any previous day in the city's history. The following morning, Mr. Jay Cooke, a leader of the city's wealthy, spoke to the press. "Few people realize we are facing a serious crisis," Cooke said. Cooke was talking about the fact that Philadelphia was lagging in its Liberty Loan Drive. Astonishingly, the *Philadelphia Inquirer* echoed Cooke's concerns. The city's sluggish bond sales could only be explained, the *In-*

quirer suggested, by the fact that it was "engaged almost to the last household in caring for the sick."

Patriotism remained hardly less infectious than Spanish influenza during the fall of 1918. Americans remained wildly—some might say insanely—patriotic during this most feverish of times. News broke. The Germans had asked President Wilson for an armistice to end the war. Headlines roared. The A.E.F. was triumphant. "Our front from the Argonne to Meuse is ablaze and the sky is lighted up by the constant glow from hundreds and hundreds of guns, speaking without cessation." Patriotism reached a fever-pitch. Many Americans opposed a negotiated end to the war; surely, it was better to let the A.E.F. simply demolish the Huns. Samuel Gompers, founder of the American Federation of Labor, protested an armistice. Massachusetts Senator Henry Cabot Lodge lamented "the sudden plunge of the Administration for a negotiated peace." In cities across the nation, Liberty Loan fever continued to burn. On October 12, President Wilson led twenty-five thousand cheering New Yorkers down the "Avenue of the Allies." That week, twenty-one hundred New Yorkers died of influenza. Liberty Loan fever burned in Philadelphia, too. At precisely 7 P.M. on October 11, church bells rang and factory whistles whined all over the city. "Town criers" in colonial dress, Boy Scouts waving Old Glory, and Liberty Bond salesmen swarmed through Philadelphia's neighborhoods. A "crier" shamed and glorified his neighbors:

> OYEZ! OYEZ! OYEZ! All who have bought Fourth Liberty Bonds shall put your four-stripe honor flag in your window before tomorrow night! If your neighbor has none, ask him why! Buy now and show your colors!
>
> FAKER! FAKER! FAKER! Why did Kaiser make his fake peace bid? To get you to weaken on this loan. Will you listen to him? No. Buy more bonds!

Like the nation as a whole, Philadelphia responded. On October 19, the final day of the Fourth Liberty Loan Drive, the nation surpassed its quota. The U.S. Secretary of the Treasury called the Drive: "The largest flotation of bonds ever made in a single effort anywhere or at any time." Remarkably, "any time" occurred in the deadliest month of America's deadliest season of plague. Senator Thompson, a Kansas Democrat touring France, wired home. The doughboys were victorious. The A.E.F. was just what was needed to "put pep into the war" and "start the ball rolling toward Berlin."

In Europe, the fall rains had begun. Despite Senator Thompson's assessment, few things were "rolling" in the Western Front. Most everything was mired in mud.

The relentless maelstrom of Meuse-Argonne continued. In the gassy, muddy trenches of the Front, men fought and slept in the rain, wearing soggy boots and clothes that never dried. Transport vehicles were scarce, and many of those were mired in the mud. Soldiers often functioned as pack mules, marching up to twenty-five kilometers a day, dragging machine-gun carts and wagons of supplies, an average of 250 pounds per man. The sick or wounded were carried on stretchers for miles through knee-deep mud, then loaded onto trucks which slowly navigated all but impassable roads to deposit their wards in damp, cold stone shelters, whatever remained of bomb-cratered French villages. U.S. Major Emerson Gillford Taylor later recalled the appalling conditions at the Front:

> Flooded dugouts, hillsides which were merely quagmires, broken roads, great difficulty in providing or procuring sufficient hot food, continually wet clothes and blankets all tended to sap the strength of the battalions posted in the gas-drenched hollows or on the slopes which were swept at all hours by snipers and artillery.

The chaplain of New York's "Fighting 69th" described his men as "dirty, lousy, thirsty, often hungry; and nearly every last man is sick." On September 23, the *Weekly Bulletin of Disease* chastised the A.E.F.'s medical officers, saying, "A man is entitled to at least the devoted care given a horse." Most doughboys would have agreed. To many disheartened soldiers, "A.E.F." (American Expeditionary Force) really stood for "Ass End First."

In September, thirty-seven thousand American and twenty-five thousand French soldiers fell sick with influenza. In October, during the second phase of the Meuse-Argonne offensive, the number climbed still higher. The Spanish Lady had become the soldier's bedfellow. To generals on both sides of the conflict, influenza was far costlier than mere numbers implied. Influenza was, quite simply, costlier than death. The dead required much less attention than the feverishly half-alive. At St. Aigan sur Cher, a busy A.E.F. transit station (which had earned the nicknames "The Mill" and "Saint Agony"), one third of those who fell sick with influenza developed secondary pneumonia; 20 to 45 percent of those who developed pneumonia died.

On October 17, Dr. George Washington Crile, a surgeon with Mobile Hospital Number 5, recorded in his diary:

> Everything is overflowing with patients. Our divisions are being shot up; the wards are full of machine-gun wounds. There is rain, mud, "flu," and pneumonia. Some hospitals are overcrowded, some are not even working. Evacuation 114 had no medical officer but hundreds of pneumonias and no one to look after them. A few days ago Major Draper asked me to see the situation with him. Every sort of infectious case was there, packed in as close as sardines with no protection. An ophthalmologist was in charge of these hundreds of cases of desperate pneumonia that are dying by the score.
>
> I have been operating on twelve-hour shifts here. One hun-

dred and twenty cases are waiting for operation this morning. In one night I had sixty deaths.

Rain, rain; mud, blood; blood, death! All day, all night we hear the incessant tramp of troops—troops going in, wounded coming back. Even in our dreams we hear it. If it ceases for a few hours, it is so insistent in our conditioned brains that the incessant rhythmic tramp continues.

The devastation Spanish influenza was wreaking on the Allied Forces gave German General Erich von Ludendorff brief cause for hope. On October 1, Ludendorff lunched with Kaiser Wilhelm. The Kaiser shared Ludendorff's optimism. Certainly influenza would sap the Allies of sufficient strength to cost them victory. Such dreams were short-lived, however. Spanish influenza was felling soldiers on both sides of the Hindenburg Line. The German army was exhausted. Ludendorff recorded in his diary: "A tired man succumbs to contagion more easily than a vigorous man." There were simply no vigorous young men, no reserves left in the embattled Rhineland.

At the end of October, Prince Max of Baden, Imperial Chancellor of Germany, the champion of and spokesman for an armistice, fell sick with flu. The Princess Blucher later described her husband's illness as part of the bizarre tragicomedy of war:

> Picture, for instance, Prince Max, a man on whose every word the whole world is waiting, lying in bed in a high state of fever, and his worried A.D.C. [aide de camp] going in and out on tiptoe, anxiously trying to extract an answer on matters of burning importance.

In Denver, Katherine Anne Porter's romance was cut short.

Like Porter herself, Miranda in "Pale Horse, Pale Rider" fell sick. Miranda's landlady nervously stopped her in the hall.

> "My dear *child*," [her landlady] said sharply, "what is the matter?" Miranda said, "Influenza, I think." "*Horrors*," said Miss Hobbe, in a whisper, and the tray wavered in her hands. "Go back to bed at once…go at *once!*"

Mild delirium and post-influenzal depression have always been well-known features of the flu. A soaring body temperature wreaks havoc on the mind. Pain, fitful sleep, ennui, sweaty chills, and fiery, parched dehydration take their toll. Convalescence can take weeks. Memory of the illness often includes little more than an odd, disquieting sense of a time unhinged from time, a bed stripped of familiarity, caretakers imbued with ghostly purpose, and wakefulness permeated with dreams and nightmares.

The bizarre physical symptoms associated with Spanish influenza were rivaled by equally bizarre effects on victims' minds. Patients were falling into hypnotic trances, experiencing vivid hallucinations, and developing amnesia. A sick postman from Norristown, Pennsylvania, "awoke" in Marlboro, Massachusetts, 250 miles from home; he never remembered how or why he had traveled there. In Minneapolis, patients of Dr. William Jones were imagining themselves powerful players on the world stage, especially the leaders of Europe's rival nations. Other delusions resembled the weird, psychedelic hallucinations of narcotic-induced trances: wallpaper writhed in sinewy designs, monkeys or spiders scuttled across beds, and snakes coiled and lunged. In Edenton, North Carolina, Sue Jordan pleaded for a place on one of the *Titanic's* lifeboats. In Dickens, Iowa, Gertie Belle Damon could not, by screaming, thrashing, or exhortations, rid her room of Kaiser Wilhelm. In Wisconsin, Lina Davis rejoiced at the nightly recital of choral music sung by her (dead) grandfather, her father, and two strangers. In Foxworth Hospital, Liverpool, sick soldiers fastened razor-blades to broom handles and fought pitched battles in the halls. And all over the world, the sick were committing suicide. Crazed patients leapt from hospital windows, bridges, and the ledges of buildings. In Washington, D.C., a thirty-six-year-old telephone employee, Alexander Reynolds, slashed his throat, then jumped out the window to his death. In Paris, the number of suicides had tripled. Volunteers patrolled the suicide-plagued Seine bridges; two volunteers, sick with flu, plunged from the Pont de la Concorde to their death.

Given the increasing panic and chaos, the hopelessness and fear, logic often became difficult to distinguish from illogic. Even for the wakeful and the well, the danger was everywhere, nowhere, vanished, imminent. The contagion was born with a breath, borne on air. Perhaps the enemy was air itself. People began blockading their houses against air: sometimes fresh air, sometimes just air itself. Windows were nailed shut. Doors were draped with heavy curtains. Oxygen-guzzling kerosene heaters blazed. Residents of Hong Kong's sweltering slums sealed windows and ventilation ducts with rags. In Citerno, Italy, a woman pressed cottonwool between the slats of her shutters and died as much of suffocation as influenza. A doctor in Waterbury, Connecticut, arrived at the home of an immigrant family to find a girl gasping for breath in a sealed room, beneath a mountain of blankets, her fever obviously self-induced. In Jamaica, islanders were sealing even the key-holes of their rooms and suffocating to death.

The residents of Meadow, Utah, were terrified. Lee Reay remembers:

> No one had ever seen the germs of the disease. No one knew where the germs were coming from. We only knew the germs

were carried by air and had gotten inside our house. We plugged up the keyholes with cotton so air couldn't get in, sealed the doors and the cracks around the doors because we thought the outside air was contaminated. One particular family, I remember, closed up every possible avenue of letting fresh air into the house. They even closed the damper on the stove. They plugged up keyholes on the door, sealed windows, and stayed inside, rebreathing their own air.

In the country town of Max Meadows, Virginia, the wife and four children of sharecropper John Brinkley were feverish with influenza and heat. Explaining that "A little fresh air could be fatal," Brinkley sealed his family in the living room around a blazing wood-stove. For seven days, Brinkley frantically fed the stove. On the eighth day, the house caught fire. Forced to remove the invalids to a vegetable patch, Brinkley despaired, "All that air will surely hasten death." But sixteen-year-old Roy Brinkley never forgot that first, heady gasp of fresh air, and the sight of cabbages looming "two feet off the ground and as big as wash tubs." Brinkley's entire family recovered. The exodus to the vegetable patch had probably saved their lives.

While physicians did not doubt the necessity of air itself, debate raged between advocates of a "fresh air" cure and closeted sickrooms. Like the fearful, bewildered public, many doctors considered fresh air an enemy of health. But there was a rising chorus of dissent. Anecdotal evidence seemed to support the medicinal value of fresh air. In Halifax, Yorkshire, a doctor smashed the sealed window of a cottage with a rolling-pin and the gasping breaths of three flu victims began to normalize. In Alberta, Canada, a physician treated influenza victims in tents pitched on hayracks. Not one patient died. Even in chilly November, the sick languishing in the courtyard of Milan's Ospedale Maggiore were more likely to recover than those in the hospital's wards. Dr. Frants Djorup pleaded with the citizens of Frederiksberg, Denmark, to remove the windows from their houses. Dr. Leonard Hill of London Hospital's Medical School suggested all British citizens sleep in the open air. Hill was convinced that cool air increased blood-flow to the membranous linings of the lungs and aided the cleansing flows which rid the blood of bacterial toxins. Too, he conjectured, cool air helped speed evaporation of the lungs' fluids—fluids in which many patients were literally drowning.

In the United States, children at New York City's Roosevelt Hospital were being given the "roof treatment." Nestled on the hospital's roof and screened from a fierce northwest wind, they were bedded down with hot water bottles and left to recover in the cold, salty air. In Massachusetts, six hospitals followed suit. The public was outraged; the treatment was labeled "barbarous and cruel." But fresh air and sunshine seemed to cause a significant drop in a patient's fever. In early October, as Boston's hospitals overflowed, Dr. Louis Croke removed 351 desperately-ill sailors to a tent community on breezy Corey Hill. Despite a week of torrential rain and crude, improvised procedures—water drawn from fire hydrants, patients kept warm with hot bricks bundled in newspaper, and, in place of non-existent face masks, gravy-strainers padded with medicated gauze—only thirty-five of Corey Hill's 351 patients died. By comparison, in Boston's hospitals, half of all influenza patients were dying.

Lee Reay's father William rode up one morning to a nearby Indian village. The Pahvant Indians, members of the Ute tribe, were camped six miles up the road from Meadow, Utah, at the edge of a canyon.

My father, being Meadow's Health Officer, was very concerned about the Indians. Nobody had gone up there to see how they were doing until my dad and the city Marshall, George Bushnell, rode up one day. My dad and Mr. Bushnell were horrified. After an Indian died, his family and friends would sit around him in a circle and chant him to the Happy Hunting Grounds. They'd chant all night long and, by the time it was over, everybody had the flu. There were lots of dead bodies in tents and families sitting around dead bodies, moaning and groaning and singing and chanting.

The first thing Dad and Mr. Bushnell did was to move all the dead bodies into three tents; then they sewed the doors shut. No one was well enough to dig graves, so my father said he'd bring up some men up from Meadow to do that. The Indians were moaning, "Medicine, medicine, medicine." The Medicine Man was sick. Dad and Mr. Bushnell asked the Chief (who was so sick he could hardly talk) if they could bring up some medicine from Meadow.

But Meadow's only doctor was sick with influenza. So William Reay decided to brew up some medicine of his own. He and George Bushnell went over to Aunt Martha Adams' house.

Aunt Martha Adams was Meadow's medicine lady. She raised all kinds of herbs for medicine. Dad asked Aunt Martha Adams, "What can we make with your herbs that will taste like medicine and maybe do some good?" She gave him quite a few things—horehound, various other herbs. My dad brought them home and stewed them up in our five-gallon washboiler. He added lots of other things, like bacon (in those days, we wrapped strips of raw bacon around our necks to cure a sore throat). My dad put anything in the pot he thought might help. And we cooked it up and it smelled like medicine and it tasted like medicine and we put in a lot of honey so it would taste good. Then we bottled it and put a label on it, "The In-fluenza Medicine." It wasn't real medicine, of course, but it made people feel better, because they thought it was medicine.

We took the medicine up to the Indian camp. I had to argue with Dad to make him let me go with him. He finally said, "You can go if you'll hold the horses and stay in the buggy. Don't come into any of the houses, but we need somebody to hold the horses so they won't walk away with the medicine." So that's what I did. I went up with them and I held the horses. I watched the Indians drink our influenza medicine and the men from Meadow dig graves.

Newspapers in Berlin were reporting that corpses were "heaped" in America's streets. In Philadelphia, at least, this seemed true.

Father Corrigan's carts still rattled through the stricken city, collecting the dead. Dr. Wilmer Krusen addressing the city's women said, "It is the duty of every well woman who can possibly get away from her other duties to volunteer for this emergency." Like women all over the country, thousands responded. Leaving their routines, their homes, and often their neighborhoods be-hind, Philadelphia's women ventured into a dangerous, chaotic world. They worked as nurses' aids, laundresses, ambulance driv-ers, and cleaning women. They ladled soup, sewed shrouds, made masks, consoled the bereaved, and closed the eyes of the dead. Only one thing was certain. To work with the sick meant putting oneself at grave risk. Still, thousands of Philadelphians volun-teered, coming to the aid of friend and stranger alike.

Clubs and private organizations pitched in. Christian par-ishes and Jewish synagogues, and political, literary, and social clubs donated time and space, creating emergency hospitals, soup kitchens, and volunteer nurse and ambulance corps. The

Philopatrian Club, a Catholic literary society, was converted into a hospital; cots were placed among shelves of musty books and Sisters of the Order of Saint Joseph, normally a monastic order, nursed the ill. Volunteers from the St. Vincent de Paul Society dug graves. Members of the Patrolmen's Benevolent Association carried bodies. Hundreds of businesses in the stricken slums of South Philadelphia distributed free food. The Philadelphia chapter of the American Red Cross donated 54,038 masks, 20,444 sheets, 8,919 towels, and 605 pairs of pajamas. The Red Cross also provided ambulances, as did the Automobile Club of Philadelphia, the Highways Transportation Committee of the National Council of Defense, and the Auto Committee of the Fourth Liberty Loan Drive.

The Philadelphia Council of National Defense coordinated the effort. Like Washington, D.C., and other cities across the nation, Philadelphia was divided into self-contained districts. Each district claimed its own medical personnel and resources. Flow in and out of hospitals was coordinated by police. An empty hospital bed was quickly filled with a patient from a list of the acutely ill. Nurses were coordinated by the Emergency Aid Nursing Committee and the Visiting Nurses Association. Each day, nurses and volunteers were distributed to the city's seven districts according to need. On October 19, Philadelphia began shooting her own version of medicine's "magic bullet" into the arms of her citizens.

In Susanna Turner's neighborhood in North Philadelphia, the parish school had been converted into an emergency hospital. The hospital was staffed by nuns, volunteers, and two Irish-women who had set up a kitchen in the basement.

I was seventeen years old and I thought I might like to be a nurse. So I went to our pastor and I asked what I could do. He told me to see Mrs. Thomas (the wife of Ira Thomas who was

the catcher for the Philadelphia *Athletics*, our city's baseball
team) who was making masks in a little side room of the hospital. Mrs. Thomas made me dip a mask in a disinfectant outside the sickroom. Then I put it on and went in. I carried bed
pans, helped the Sisters the best I could. People were so
weak, they almost seemed dead.

Every once in a while, I'd stiffen up and get scared and wonder if I was going to get the flu. But I was surviving. I just lived
from day to day. I didn't think about the future.

Still, despite the efforts of Susanna Turner and thousands
like her, Philadelphia's most gruesome problem remained.
Corpses were everywhere. The customary rituals surrounding
death—care of the deceased, wake, burial, and ceremonies of
remembrance and faith—became a luxury few could afford and
public health officials could not allow.

Five supplementary morgues were opened. Ten embalmers
were begged from the Secretary of War. Police joined others in
combing the city for the dead. Convicts were made to dig graves.
The Bureau of Highways continued to gouge trenches in Potter's
Field with a steam shovel; trenches were dug in cemeteries all
over Philadelphia. Complaints arose: undertakers were raising
prices by 600 percent and cemetery officials were charging fifteen dollars for burial and sometimes even making the bereaved
relatives dig graves. In truth, undertakers were overwhelmed;
they were no more unscrupulous, no more immune to the mercenary laws of supply and demand which had led even Washington's Commissioner Louis Brownlow to hijack a shipment of
coffins. Many had rendered services for which they had not been
paid. Given the scope of the crisis, the lack of embalmers, and
scarcity of coffins, many undertakers simply could not afford to
accept more bodies without payment. In recognition of this, the
Council of National Defense hired local woodworkers to make

"simple pine boxes" to be used only for Philadelphians. Undertakers were allowed to add only 20 percent to the cost. Philadelphia's mayor guaranteed undertakers would be paid for all services rendered with city funds.

The crisis in Philadelphia was replayed throughout the nation and the world. Those in coffins were the lucky ones. "All a boy got when he died was a winding sheet," Nurse Josie Mabel Brown remembered. "We just couldn't get enough caskets." In Boston, an immigrant named Leo Lafieri left the body of his two-year-old on a back shelf at a mortuary; he simply did not have the money to pay for a casket. It was five days before the small corpse was discovered. Plagued by shortages, the city of Buffalo, like Philadelphia, began making its own coffins. Health commissioner Dr. Frankin C. Gram announced, "They will not be one thousand dollar caskets, or even one hundred dollar caskets. They will be plain and respectable." In Japan, coffins were being fashioned from sake barrels, cardboard, and paper. In Central Europe, coffins were virtually unobtainable; the dead were buried in sheets or nothing at all. In Germany, coffins were being sold on the black market or briefly loaned for the journey to the cemetery.

In Athens, Greece, bodies lay unburied for days. In Norway, where the earth was frozen, the dead were simply strung in trees to await the spring thaw.

The Donohues' small neighborhood funeral home in West Philadelphia was overwhelmed. The modern, motorized hearse, proudly engraved with the family name, could not keep up. The slow creak of the funeral wagon was heard once again.

> Everything was in panic, disarray. We were burying our neighbors, our friends, people we did business with, people we went

to church with. The bodies never stopped coming. The sadness, the heartbreak went on and on, day after day.

To Michael Donohue, the spectacle of bereaved relatives digging graves for their loved ones was a sad but inevitable consequence of the crisis.

The cemeteries went to extraordinary lengths to help people, especially the Archdiocese of Philadelphia. In some cases, families had to dig the graves themselves, but it was either that or they weren't going to get the grave open. In order to maintain some level of humanity, the Archdiocese brought in a steam shovel to excavate section 42 of Holy Cross Cemetery—what became known as the "trench." The trench was the cemetery's way of expediting burials to help families, give people closure. They lined up the dead, one right after another, and did the committal prayers right there in the trench.

The Donohues' ledger books date back to 1898. They contain a vivid record of 1918's chaotic October:

Our ledger books are all handwritten and the ones from 1918 are written in the flowing fancy penmanship common in that era. In the early part of 1918, things are well documented. You can tell who a person was, who his parents were, his children. The book lists where he lived, what he died of, where the viewing and funeral were held, where he was buried. But when you get to October 1918, the ledgers become sloppy and confused; things are crossed out, scribbled in borders. Information is scant and all out of chronological order—it's nearly impossible to keep track of what's going on, it's just page after page of tragedy and turmoil. Sometimes we got paid. Sometimes we didn't. Usually, we buried people we knew. Other times, we buried strangers. One entry reads, "A girl." Another says "A Polish woman." Another: "A Polish man and his baby." Someone must have asked us to take care of these people and it was just the decent thing to do. We had a responsibility to make sure things were done in a proper, moral, dignified manner. Scribbled at the bottom of the ledger, below the entry for the "girl," is "This girl was buried in the trench." This girl was our addition to the trench. I guess we had nowhere else to put her.

Usually a mortician sees people dying in their forties, their fifties, some older, some in their nineties. But in the fall of 1918, young people were dying: eighteen-year-olds, twenty-year-olds, thirty-year-olds, forty-year-olds. These were people who should not have died. Most of them were either first generation immigrants or right from their countries of origin: Ireland or Poland or Italy. These were people who came to the Promised Land. They came to start fresh, and when they got here, their lives were destroyed.

In Philadelphia's Rittenhouse Square, the doleful peals of the funeral bells continued. Columba Voltz's parents had fallen sick. Neither her father nor mother could move from bed. She remembers:

> I was petrified. I was only eight. I didn't know what to do. None of our relatives would come near us for fear of getting sick. And all day long, those horrible funeral bells rang: BONG, BONG, BONG. I heard them even in my sleep.

In "Pale Horse, Pale Rider," Miranda drifts in and out of consciousness. "Let's sing," she says to Adam. "I know an old spiritual." She begins in a hoarse whisper, "Pale horse, pale rider, done taken my lover away..."

In 1918, Mary McCarthy was growing up in Seattle. Like Katherine Anne Porter, McCarthy would become a celebrated writer. In 1918, she was six, one of four children. Her parents, Roy and Tess, were a dashing, handsome couple. McCarthy never forgot the Seattle of that terrible autumn. She later wrote:

> No hospital beds were to be had, and people went about with masks, or stayed shut up in their houses...the awful fear of contagion made each man an enemy to his neighbor.

At the end of October, the McCarthy family boarded a train east. Their destination was Minneapolis, home of Roy's parents.

> I remember sitting beside my father on that train trip and looking out the window at the Rocky Mountains. All the rest of the party are lying sick in bed in their compartments, and I am feeling proud of the fact that my father and I are still well, riding upright in that Pullman car. As we look up at the mountains, my father tells me that big boulders sometimes fell off them, hitting the train and killing people. Listening, I start to shake and my teeth to chatter with what I think is terror but what turns out to be the flu.

Of London in 1355, during the Black Death, Daniel Defoe wrote:

> Many houses were then left desolate, all the people being carried away dead.... there were several houses together which... had not one person left alive in them, and some that died last in several of those houses were left a little too long before they

were fetched out to be buried; the reason of which was not, as some have written very untruly, that the living were not sufficient to bury the dead, but that the mortality was so great in the yard or alley that there was nobody left to give notice to the buriers or sextons that there were any dead bodies to be buried.... The dead carts were several times, as I have heard, found standing by the churchyard gate full of dead bodies, but neither bellman or driver or any one else with it.

In a small room above a tailor's shop in Philadelphia, a neighbor had arrived to nurse Columba Voltz's parents. Columba tried to help. "I made mustard plasters and put them on my parents' chests. I brought lemonade, ran errands." Still, Columba was drawn to the front window of the apartment. She watched the grim ebb and flow of coffins, the unending funerals moving swiftly in and out of the parish church. At first, Columba was not sure she was sick. Perhaps she was just sad. Her teeth started chattering. Pain shot through her head. She felt a dizzy, feverish heat. She crawled into bed.

All I heard was those horrible bells: BONG, BONG, BONG. I was terrified. I was too afraid even to move. I lay very still, almost without breathing. All day long, I heard those funeral bells. I was sure I was going to die. I was sure they were going to put me inside a coffin, and carry me inside the church. I was sure those horrible bells were going to ring for me.

Chapter 7

Horror

In Denver, Colorado, Katherine Anne Porter's flu led to delirium. Her fever became so high her hair turned white and fell out. Her lieutenant nursed her patiently, despite the shrill objections of her landlady. From "Pale Horse, Pale Rider":

> Miss Hobbe with her face all out of shape with terror was crying shrilly, "I tell you they must come for her now, or I'll put her on the sidewalk...I tell you, this is a plague, a plague, my God!"
>
> I lay back on the pillow and thought, I must give up, I can't hold out any longer. There was only that pain, only that room. There was only this one moment and it was a dream of time... "I'm not unconscious," I explained, "I know what I want to say." Then to my horror I heard myself babbling nonsense...
>
> A terrible compelling pain ran through her veins like heavy fire. The stench of corruption filled her nostrils, the sweetish sickening smell of rotting flesh and pus. The smell of death was in her own body.

All across the nation, men, women, and children were sick. For millions of Americans, life had become a painful, nightmarish ordeal. For the robust, those who remained standing, life had become nearly as surreal. All health seemed vanished from the world. The plague was everywhere. No city, no home, no family,

153

no person was safe. Like the medieval Black Death, Spanish influenza was as implacable and ephemeral as fog, an oppressive, ghostly presence. According to schoolgirl Georgina Cragg, "the fear was so thick even a child could feel it." The rituals of community life—gossip over the pushcart, conversation by the fence-post, the games of children and the commerce of churches—all the discrete moments which, woven together, created the rich fabric of American life—were failing to occur. Even an act as simple and natural as shaking hands could invite the angel of death. People were afraid of each other. Neighbors vanished inside their homes. Life had been utterly disrupted.

In the Sardo's funeral home in Washington, D.C., the fear was palpable. Bill Sardo remembers:

> From the moment I got up in the morning to when I went to bed at night, I felt a constant sense of fear. We wore gauze masks. We were afraid to kiss each other, to eat with each other, to have contact of any kind. We had no family life, no school life, no church life, no community life. Fear tore people apart.

In Philadelphia, Susanna Turner's neighborhood had turned into a bleak, unwelcoming place.

> Neighbors weren't helping neighbors. No one was taking any chances. People became selfish. We lost our spirit of charity. Fear just withered the hearts of people.

Dan Tonkel of Goldsboro, North Carolina recalls:

> I felt like I was walking on eggshells. I was afraid to go out, to play with my playmates, my classmates, my neighbors. I was almost afraid to breathe. I remember I was actually afraid to breathe. People were afraid to talk to each other. It was like—

don't breathe in my face, don't even look at me, because you
might give me germs that will kill me.

The peaceful rhythms of small town life had been shattered.
Goldsboro's streets were deserted.

> Farmers stopped farming, merchants stopped selling. The
> county more or less just shut down. Everyone was holding their
> breath, waiting for something to happen. So many people were
> dying, we could hardly count them. We never knew from one
> day to another who was going to be next on the death list.

All across America, community life was grinding to a halt.
Schools and factories closed. Churches, libraries, and private
clubs locked their doors. Courts recessed. Newspapers folded or
simply stopped printing ("Don't expect the next *Courier* until you
see it," one wrote). Government services failed. Policemen were
sick, as were firemen, trash collectors, and trolley drivers. Garbage
remained dumped on city streets. No "Operator" answered to
place a call. Essentials, like food and coal, became scarce: mer-
chants were sick or fearful. Steel and coal production faltered, as
did the machinery and business of war. Riveting guns fell silent in
naval shipyards. Production lines halted in munitions factories.
Army camps were paralyzed. Army Chief of Staff Payton March
cabled General Pershing in France, "Influenza not only stopped
all draft calls in October, but practically all training."

The business of war and the commerce of daily life in America were both falling victim to the plague. Captain George T.
Palmer of the Army Sanitary Corps advised, "Abandon the uni-
versal practice of shaking hands. Substitute some other less inti-
mate method of salutation." Americans were cautioned against
leaving home, against riding trolleys, against checking a book out
from the library, against "slacking" with their masks. The maga-

zine *Science* reported 119 daily opportunities for infection, from turning a doorknob to paying a grocery bill. Official and unofficial advice poured forth, intensifying the dread and panic, feeding a mad rumor-mill of weird, improbable cures and contradictory advice. Castor oil was advisable. Castor oil was not advisable. Fresh air and exercise were the ticket; it was better to stay home and rest. No one knew what to do.

Widespread rumors of a German plot intensified. Some claimed Bayer aspirin (whose original patent had been German) was filled with poisoned germs. The Public Health Service was compelled to investigate the claims, claims which were disproved. Had German spies infiltrated the Army Medical Corps and spread Spanish influenza through hypodermic shots? Had the spies had been discovered and executed by firing squad? Rumors persisted, despite strenuous denials by the Surgeon General of the Army, Brigadier General Charles Richard: "There have been no medical officers or nurses or anyone else executed at camps in the United States." Nevertheless, many Americans continued to blame the Germans for Spanish influenza. One patriot declared,

> Let the curse be called the German plague. Let every child learn to associate what is accursed with the word German not in the spirit of hate but in the spirit of contempt born of the hateful truth which Germany has proved herself to be.

The moral fabric of America was unraveling, bit by bit. The foundations of American society—education, law, religion—all seemed in jeopardy. Even the institution of family was shaken. Influenza was the invisible enemy. The visible enemy, the clear and obvious source of danger, was one's fellow man—especially the members of one's family. Many families, out of necessity, lack of options, love, compassion, or feelings of dutiful responsibility, persisted in what was, at the time, a familiar exercise: to nurse

one's own. Because of the breadth of the catastrophe, women, society's traditional "ministering angels," were joined in great numbers by men like Katherine Anne Porter's gentle lieutenant and
William Maxwell's grim uncle. For other families, however, the
silent, savage intruder which had invaded their home, their dinner table, and their beds exposed or aggravated existing tensions.
Often, answering a call reporting the terminally ill, health authorities would arrive at the scene and find no one home but the
dying—the families had deserted them. In Minneapolis, a hundred homeless children, some sick, some not, were found hiding
out on the streets, their parents vanished.

In West Philadelphia, every hour brought another knock on
the door of the Donohues' funeral home from people bearing
their dead. Increasingly, the grim pandemonium contained a
bizarre irony. Desperate to provide dignity for their deceased
relatives, people were stealing caskets. The Donohues were
forced to hire men to guard their small stash of coffins. Michael
Donohue explains:

> Normally, stealing a casket would be inconceivable. It would
> be equated with grave robbing. But in October 1918, the in-
> fluenza epidemic changed people's minds about what they
> would do, how they would act. People were desperate. They
> felt they had no alternative, there was no place for them to
> turn. These were nice people, people who wouldn't have done
> this otherwise. These were our neighbors, our friends, and for
> some of them, stealing a casket was the only way they could see
> to provide for their loved one.

Autumn had truly become the season of death.

The numbers were staggering. In the state of New York,
500,000 people were sick with influenza and related pneumonia. In Pennsylvania, 350,000 were sick; in New Jersey,

100,000; Connecticut, 110,000; Virginia, 220,000; Ohio, 150,000; Nebraska, 40,000; Minnesota, 35,000; and California, 40,000. In Venice, California, the Al. G. Barnes Circus underwent a mandatory "fumigation." Lions, elephants, and ponies, as well as trapeze artists, contortionists, and the "Albino Girl," were sprayed with a foul mixture of coal tar and formaldehyde. In Chicago, October 17 became known as "Black Thursday": 381 people died and 1,200 fell sick. The city ran out of hearses. Passenger trolleys were draped in black and used to collect bodies. Signs were posted:

> There shall be no public funerals held in Chicago over any body dead from any disease or cause whatsoever. No wakes or public gatherings of any kind shall be held in connection with these bodies. No one except adult relatives and friends not to exceed ten persons in addition to the undertaker, undertaker's assistants, minister, and necessary drivers shall be permitted to attend any funeral. No dead body shall be taken into any church or chapel for funeral services in connection with such body.

Laws veered towards the brutal. Chicago's Health Commissioner, Dr. John Dill Robertson, turned his considerable wrath against spitters and "openfaced sneezers." He ordered the police, "Arrest thousands, if necessary, to stop sneezing in public!" Only Reverend J.P. Brushingham of Chicago's Morals Commission noted a silver lining in the plague's dark cloud. In the month of October, Chicago's crime rate dropped by 43 percent.

Even New York's nervy, indomitable Royal Copeland was growing tense. Each day, 5,500 New Yorkers fell sick with influenza. On October 23, 851 people died: mortality figures which surpassed even those of Philadelphia. The Empire City and the Empire State had become the deadliest place in the nation.

Health Commissioner Copeland, whose rambling and verbose Congressional oratories later earned him the nickname "General Exodus," lashed out at his fellow physicians. Sloppy morbidity and mortality reports were skewing the daily totals. Late or messy reports would be slapped with a five hundred dollar fine. State Commissioner of Health, Herman Biggs, joined in with a fine of his own: any person who coughed or sneezed in the state of New York without a handkerchief would pay five hundred dollars or spend a year in jail. Huge signs appeared on New York streets: "It is Unlawful to Cough and Sneeze." Five hundred "snifflers" were dragged into court. Spitters suffered a similar fate.

In Brooklyn, New York, six-year-old Michael Wind stood among his brothers and sisters.

> When my mother died of Spanish influenza, we were all gathered in one room, all six of us, from age two to age twelve. My father was sitting beside my mother's bed, head in his hands, sobbing bitterly. All my mother's friends were there, with tears of shock in their eyes. They were shouting at my father, asking why he hadn't called them, hadn't told them she was sick. She had been fine yesterday. How could this have happened?

The next morning, his father took Michael and his two younger brothers to the subway. He bought each child a Hershey bar. Michael Wind: "I knew then that something was wrong. My father couldn't afford such treats. Sure enough, we were on our way to an orphanage." Michael and his brothers were placed in the Brooklyn Hebrew Orphan Asylum. The Asylum was filled with six hundred boys and girls, most orphaned by the flu.

Flamboyant Evangelist Billy Sunday continued to preach and

"pray down" the plague. In October, he turned his forceful attentions west. San Francisco, Sunday declared, was "going to hell so fast it ought to be arrested for speeding." Indeed, one quarter of California's forty thousand sick were in San Francisco.

San Francisco had mobilized with incredible unity. The entire city had donned masks; the Red Cross had pumped vaccine into thousands of arms. But as the crisis deepened, even Dr. William Hassler, chief of San Francisco's Board of Health and a seasoned public health official, floundered. Like officials across the nation, Hassler divided his city into self-contained districts, each claiming its own resources. Hassler divided San Francisco into twenty districts, then nine, then fourteen, then twelve. Venturing one day down Grant Street into the labyrinthine heart of the city's crammed, insular Chinatown, Hassler was appalled at the sight of influenza victims languishing in close quarters, fearful of and unresponsive to official "help." Hassler could do little more than advise wealthy San Franciscans to keep their Asian servants in their own homes and away from Chinatown.

The genteel city was feeling the strain. Dental students were serving as doctors. Schoolteachers were working as laundresses. Paddy-wagons had become ambulances and policemen were collecting bodies. The entire staff of the coroner's office was down with influenza and a fireman was running the morgue. Terrified San Franciscans suggested that the Pacific be pumped through city hydrants to continually flush the streets. Mayor Rolph responded helplessly, "You might as well sit out and watch the changes of the moon."

On the morning of October 18, Mrs. Sarah Doyle appeared in municipal court to sue her husband for divorce. Mr. Doyle arrived, announcing he had influenza and had just crawled out of bed. Mr. Doyle's attorney fled. The judge appointed two more attorneys in quick succession, but they ran away, too, as did everyone in the courtroom except the judge and the Doyles. Mr. Doyle became argumentative. The judge turned him over to the sheriff, who handed him over the Board of Health.

A package arrived at William Hassler's office: "Compliments of John." The package contained three pounds of gunpowder with buckshot and broken glass, attached to a crude timing device. "John" was no doubt protesting Hassler's emergency ordinances, probably mask-wearing. In fact, the San Francisco Red Cross had run out of masks. "Mask-profiteering" had begun. Still, Hassler maintained that the scarcity of masks was no excuse for lapsing with the "gauze." A Health Department inspector shot a blacksmith who refused to wear a mask. Two innocent bystanders were caught in the crossfire. A taxi driver, W.S. Tickner, picked up three mask-wearing passengers. The men robbed Tickner at gunpoint, dumped him out of his cab and roared away, still wearing their masks as required by law. On the night of November 8, San Francisco police raided the lobbies of downtown hotels. Four hundred "mask-slackers" were arrested. The guilty, most of whom had loosened their masks to enjoy a quick smoke, were packed into paddy wagons and taken off to City Prison. The mayor of Denver, observing the melee in San Francisco, sighed: "Why, it would take half the population of our city to make the other half wear masks."

Death was everywhere. Virtually everyone in America felt threatened.

In New Mexico, armed vigilantes forced visitors from more flu-ridden places to get back on trains and return to where they had come from.

In Prescott, Arizona, it became a crime to shake hands. The town had gotten the idea from a young newspaperman in Italy— Benito Mussolini.

In Chicago, a recent immigrant named Peter Marrazo barricaded his family inside their apartment, shouting, "I'll cure them my own way!" He slashed the throats of his wife and four children. They had not been sick.

On a train headed east from Seattle, every member of Mary McCarthy's family was now sick, including Mary and her father, Roy. A conductor tried to force them off the train. Roy pulled a gun. Feverishly ill, Roy defiantly guarded his family as the train made its way slowly east, towards Minneapolis.

In Newark, New Jersey, 107,000 people were sick with flu. Newark's mayor, Charles P. Gillen, took tight hold of the reins of his besieged city. He issued a rapid-fire succession of directives, orders which confused and outraged many. Gillen made his office the sole source of information regarding the epidemic. He instituted a city-wide quarantine. He revoked the quarantine. His political opponents claimed Gillen had "lost his head." New Jersey's State Board of Health revoked Gillen's revocation and reinstated his original quarantine, stating, "The epidemic still prevails in the city of Newark to a very alarming extent." Gillen's foes, rejoicing in the Mayor's castigation, claimed Gillen had lifted the quarantine because he was tired of "sneaking through the back doors of saloons." Gillen was undaunted. Calling the State Board of Health's ruling "hysterical" and "absurd," he refused to impose a quarantine. Instead, he defiantly ordered saloons, movie houses, and other businesses to reopen. Legislators in the state capital demanded Gillen's impeachment. Nevertheless, on October 22, beer flowed once again through taps in Newark's saloons. Lights went on in movie houses. Charlie Chaplin returned in "Shoulder Arms," Theda Bara in "When a Woman Sins," and Harold Lockwood in "Pals First" (Lockwood died of influenza on October 23). Still, amid the public fracas, the private catastrophes continued. The *Newark Evening News* announced the engagement of Miss Margaret Colie of Prospect Street, East Orange, to Ensign Theodore Burnham Van Nest of Litchfield, Connecticut. The next day, the *Evening News* announced Ensign Van Nest had died of influenza on a ship bound for France. On Livingston Street in Newark, Mr. Padolek died of influenza. Some days later, a despondent Mrs. Padolek turned on the gas jets and committed suicide.

In Philadelphia, Anna Milani and all her brothers and sisters fell ill.

> The pain was awful. I remember the terrible, terrible headache, the pain all over my body, in my legs, my stomach, my chest. We were all very, very sick. Our father made us drink chamomile tea. Our mother made plasters out of flour. She couldn't afford mustard plasters, so she heated up flour, put it in a warm cloth, and put it on our chests.

Two-year-old Harry grew worse. Harry was Anna's favorite. A neighbor brought a doctor to the house. The doctor said Harry had double pneumonia.

> I was like a second mother to Harry. When Harry got sick, he called for me all the time. Even though I was sick, I was always beside him. I would cuddle and pet him; I couldn't do anything else. Harry had big, beautiful eyes, but his face got so thin, his eyes bulged out. He was in so much pain. We were all in so much pain.

In another Philadelphia neighborhood, Harriet Ferrel was sick with influenza. So were her father, brother, sister, aunt, uncle, and cousin. Harriet's mother was nursing all seven.

> Our family doctor, Dr. Milton White, came by. He told my mother she didn't need to feed me anymore, because I wasn't going to live. He said if I did live, I would be blind.

In "Pale Horse, Pale Rider," Miranda is separated from her

lover, Adam. She is taken to a hospital and Adam is not allowed to visit her. Miss Tanner, a volunteer, sits beside her bed.

"I know those are your hands," Miranda told Miss Tanner, "I know it, but to me they are white tarantulas, don't touch me."

"Shut your eyes," said Miss Tanner.

"Oh, no," said Miranda, "for then I see worse things," but her eyes closed in spite of her will, and the midnight of her internal torment closed about her...

The road to death is a long march beset with all evils, and the heart fails little by little at each new terror, the bones rebel at each step, the mind sets up its own bitter resistance and to what end....I shall not know when it happens, I shall not feel or remember, why can't I consent now, I am lost, there is no hope for me. Look, [Miranda] told herself, there it is, that is death and there is nothing to fear....Silenced, she sank easily through depths under depths of darkness until she lay like a stone at the farthest bottom of life.

In Philadelphia, Anna Milani's mother insisted she lie down.

My mother said I'd been up too long taking care of Harry. I should rest. While I was lying down, Harry died. My mother came to get me. She was crying, holding my baby sister and crying. She said Harry had opened his eyes—his head rolled back and forth—and he said, "Nanina." My name was Nanina in Italian. Harry died with my name in his mouth.

There were no embalmers, so my parents covered Harry with ice. There were no coffins, just boxes painted white. My parents put Harry in a box. My mother wanted him dressed in white—it had to be white. So she dressed him in a little white suit and put him in the box. You'd think he was sleeping. We all said a little prayer. The priest came over and blessed him.

I remember my mother putting a white piece of cloth over his face; then they closed the box. They put Harry in a little wagon, drawn by a horse. Only my father and uncle were allowed to go to the cemetery. When they got there, two soldiers lowered Harry into a hole.

The nation's wildest, most remote province braced itself. The governor of Alaska, Thomas Riggs, Jr., was well aware of the epidemic raging in the lower states, the territory known to Alaskans as the "Outside." Riggs acted swiftly. He imposed a maritime quarantine. He restricted travel to the interior. He stationed U.S. Marshals at ports of debarkation, trail heads, and the mouths of Alaska's rivers. He closed schools, churches, theaters, and pool halls. Local authorities followed Riggs' lead. In Juneau, citizens were instructed to "keep as much to yourself as possible." Fairbanks established quarantine stations, also guarded by marshals. Citizens were checked periodically for flu and given arm bands reading "O.K., Fairbanks Health Department." The wilderness hamlet of Shaktoolik reacted in grand frontier style, hiring guards "for a wage of four deer each month." Anyone who disobeyed the town's sanctions would be forced to supply the town with cords of firewood, "sawed, split, and piled." Vaccine was imported from Seattle, distributed throughout the state. Native shamans offered their own remedies. "Medicine trees" were planted in front of Eskimo villages and alongside trails.

Still, as she had the world over, the Spanish Lady defied attempts to spurn her. Exploding through quarantine stations at Nome and Juneau, she spread rapidly along the coast into the interior. Half of Nome's white population fell ill. Superintendent of Education Walter Shields, head of Alaska's teachers, critical liaisons between natives and whites, was one of the first to die. Nome's Eskimo village was decimated: 176 of 300 Eskimos died. The Arctic explorer, Vilhjalmur Stefansson, arrived in Seattle, telling a gruesome tale. Terrified and superstitious, Nome's Eskimos had raced from cabin to cabin until panic and disease infected all. Entire families, too sick to replenish fires, froze to death. Eskimos removed to a makeshift hospital, believing it was a death-house, hanged themselves. Five of Stefansson's eight Eskimo guides had died in Nome, including twenty-five-year-old Split-the-Wind, widely considered Alaska's greatest musher. During his last expedition to the Pole, Split-the-Wind and Stefansson's other guides had endured brutal conditions. To survive, they had eaten their snowshoe lacings. Now they were all dead of flu.

On November 7, Governor Riggs issued a special directive "To All Alaska Natives." Eskimos were ordered to stay home, refuse visitors, and avoid public gatherings. But Riggs' directive was an anathema to Eskimo life, which revolved around traditional rituals of communality, hospitality, and sharing. And so the panic of Nome's Eskimos was repeated in villages throughout the state. The report of a schoolteacher at Hamilton revealed the mutual misapprehensions between white and native. Initially, Hamilton's Eskimos were unconcerned about the flu, but as the village swiftly sickened, panic set in, as did superstitious terror:

> Then they refused to help themselves but preferred to sit on the floor and wait to die. I did everything for them; furnished wood and water, split kindling, made shavings, built fires, cooked food and delivered it to them, and even acted as undertaker and hearse driver. Apparently the native had no regard but rather fear for their dead. Frequently I had to rescue corpses from the dogs which began to eat them.

In Suitna, all but two of the Eskimos became sick. Katherine G. Kane, a schoolteacher from the Bureau of Indian Affairs, found victims huddled inside cabins, dying of influenza, starvation, and cold. No one was healthy enough to split firewood or harvest moose. Starving, desperately sick Eskimos were doing the unthinkable—killing and eating their sled dogs. In other villages, like Hamilton, the tables were turned. Ravenous dogs were eating the dead and dying alike.

Spanish influenza moved still further into Alaska's interior, slipped down the Seward Peninsula. Mailmen brought her to Teller, Solomon, Golovin, Mary's Igloo, York, Wales. In York, everyone died. In Wales, the 170 dead included five children who were born and died during the epidemic. A schoolteacher reported:

> Three [villages] wiped out entirely, others average 85 percent deaths.... Total number of deaths reported 750, probably 25 percent this number froze to death before help arrived. Over three hundred children to be cared for, majority of whom are orphans. Am feeding and caring for surviving population of five large villages.

In the village of Teller, the whites died first. Reverend Rosso died, then the schoolteacher, the local interpreter, and the interpreter's wife and child. Influenza engulfed the natives. Only Mrs. Rosso, the wife of the dead clergyman and mother of a newborn baby, remained to care for the village. Eighty of Teller's 150 residents died. Six miles away, in Teller Mission, 85 percent of the population perished in a single week.

On October 7, 1918, war at last conspired to separate Private John Lewis Barkley from his Cherokee Indian buddies. Barkley had met Floyd and "Jesse" James while sick with influenza in a camp hospital in Fort Riley, Kansas. Since then, the three had been inseparable.

In the gassy, murky Argonne forest, assessment of German troop movements had become nearly impossible. Sergeant Nayhone of Intelligence told Barkley, "The aviators haven't been able to find out a damned thing. Somebody's got to go." Wearily, Barkley responded, "If you want to bump me off, for God's sake do it here."

As he had so many times before, Barkley crawled and slithered through the Argonne woods. He settled within yards of the German line in a muddy bomb-crater on the slope of Hill 253. All night, Barkley huddled over his field telephone, scanning the woods for movement. The pallid dawn brought the thunder of German artillery, answered by American shells. Germans were flitting among the oaks, preparing for an attack. Barkley's phone buzzed. Sergeant Nayhone barked, "Be on your toes. Stay with it as long as you can. And take care. If anything..." The phone went dead before Barkley could warn Nayhone of the attack. But perhaps, Barkley thought, he could stall the Germans. He had seen a Maxim machine gun and several boxes of ammunition in the woods. A small French Renault tank, abandoned on a nearby ridge, was surrounded by the bloody refuse of war: bloated corpses, canteens, bread, bloody bayonets, and boxes of ammunition. American smoke shells exploded. A thick pall of dense smoke descended across the woods. Under cover of smoke, Barkley raced through the trees. Grabbing the Maxim, he sprinted towards the French tank. He gathered ammunition, slid inside. Several hundred yards away, six hundred German soldiers were advancing into an open field. Barkley opened fire. Soldiers fell. Others raced for cover. Barkley had been spotted. Even as the tank, peppered with bullets, rocked and began to smoke, Barkley continued to spray the field with machine gun fire. All afternoon, the stalemate continued: John Barkley against hundreds of Germans. Gradually, Barkley realized he was being backed up. An American sniper was methodically, deftly picking off Germans. Still, bullets screamed closer. Barkley heard a sudden ringing in his ears. Blood gushed from his nose.

Barkley's head swum. He remembered a hospital in the dusty, unforgiving badlands of Kansas and a boy in a hospital bed next to him, grabbing him with an icy, vice-like hand. All Barkley could think of was the telltale nasal hemorrhage of Spanish influenza.

When a high fever breaks suddenly, a patient can enter a state resembling shock. The fever's fiery heat (hyperthermia) is replaced by the extreme cold of hypothermia. Bodily functions slow. Cardiac and respiratory activity become nearly imperceptible. Dehydration has literally drained the body of blood; there is less blood pumping through veins and arteries, less blood to hear in the pulse or heartbeat.

In the autumn of 1918, medical personnel were overwhelmed or nonexistent. Exhausted (and often ill), doctors signed death certificates without even viewing the body. Hundreds of thousands were buried without death certificates altogether. In many places, hospitals had literally become death houses. Makeshift emergency hospitals were just that—makeshift: county jails, dance halls, hayracks. In the fall of 1918, the medical "system" had become an eclectic assortment of facilities which were at once boldly inventive and hopelessly crude. All over the world, tales were being told of the most nightmarish of medical mistakes. Whether because of hypothermia or other bedeviling complications of Spanish influenza such as coma and encephalitis (inflammation of the brain), the barely alive were sometimes confused with the dead.

In Naples, Italy, Giovanni Campanella squirmed free of his loosely-nailed coffin, terrifying the mourners who were attending his wake. An undertaker in Wellington, New Zealand, was removing Robert Coulter to a hearse, the boy's death certificate in hand, when he heard Robert "sigh"; the boy made a full recovery. In Cape Town, South Africa, Kate Le Roux watched as a truck loaded with coffins hit a pothole and lurched out of control. Coffins tumbled to the ground. One flew open. A man crawled out and scrambled down the street—a Mr. Irving, who lived to tell the horrific tale for another fifty years. In Spain, Dr. Juan Zamora, asked to issue a death certificate, decided to inspect the body first. He found the victim in a stage of illness known as "apparent death." The patient was cold as ice, without pulse or discernible respiration. His nightshirt was drenched, however, and Zamora knew he had recently been sweating a high fever. Hypothermia had slowed his heart. With massage, artificial respiration, and injections of caffeine and adrenaline, Zamora revived the "corpse."

In a parish hospital in Philadelphia, the curiosity of seventeen-year-old Susanna Turner saved the life of a woman and baby.

> Francis, a young man who ran errands, told me the pregnant lady had died. "Where is she?" I asked. Francis said, "In the back room of the school." So we walked down the hall and I said, "Francis, I think I hear a noise in there." We went in. She was alive. The nuns called the ambulance. The woman was taken to a hospital where she delivered her child.

A much more grim ending awaited a family in the Southwest. A doctor in Las Vegas, New Mexico, pronounced Clara Garduno dead. Health Department officials insisted she be buried immediately. Her sick husband, Frank, crawled from bed and begged the services of an undertaker. Three of the Garduno's children were morbidly ill, and Clara's grave was left uncovered, so the children could be buried with her. That afternoon, two of the Garduno's children died. While burying the baby, Frank asked to view his wife one last time. The coffin was opened. Clara had been buried alive. She had rolled onto her stomach, her hair tangled in her claw-like fingers.

In France, General Pershing was sick with influenza.

In suicide-plagued Paris, funerals were only allowed at night. An endless stream of hearses and horse-drawn carts rumbled along the Avenue Jean Jaurès to Pantin Cemetery.

In India, tens of thousands of bodies awaited cremation. Armageddon seemed to have arrived. Dr. M.C. Nanjunda Rau mused:

> This pandemic must [be] the result of some cosmic influence operating on the vitality of all living things, reducing their power of resistance against disease, thus rendering them easy victims to the onslaughts of many germs. Thus, this pandemic may be considered perhaps the closing era of a certain type of civilization or of a certain type of man.

Inside a bullet-pocked tank in the French Argonne, Private John Lewis Barkley regained consciousness. The violent nosebleed which had so terrified him, reminding him of the nasal hemorrhage of Spanish influenza, had been caused by a wrenching explosion. Even as grenades continued to rock the tank and Barkley let loose round after round of gunfire, he realized the Germans were retreating. Barkley's lone stand was ending. The U.S. Seventh Division swept over the crest of Hill 253. Rejoining his division, Barkley was delighted to discover that his buddy 'Jesse' James had been the sniper who had backed him up during his perilous stand.

The pact made long ago in Fort Riley, Kansas, could no longer be honored. Floyd's bullet wound had become infected. The big Cherokee fought off medics, but was lashed to a stretcher and taken away. Soon afterwards, in a barn in the Argonne woods, Barkley peeled off his muddy boots and collapsed into the hay. A fellow scout, Mike de Angelo, a featherweight boxer from Philadelphia, banged on the farmhouse door, pleading for help.

For two days, Barkley thrashed in a sweaty fever. He awoke in a plush featherbed. Curious strangers were peering at him. None of his French hosts spoke English and Barkley spoke no French. Barkley realized he was clad only in an enormous nightshirt. He later recalled, "A sturdy, good-looking young woman was trying to pour some kind of hot toddy down my throat. She was the one who'd carried me into the house." Barkley pleaded for his clothes. Madame only laughed.

> That evening the two women bathed me as if I were a baby. I made an awful fuss at first, but it didn't do a bit of good. I'd pull the sheet up over me and they'd pull it down again and go on with their work. I gave up after a while. I was so weak the girl alone could have handled me.... They gave me an alcohol rub. They washed my head and put some kind of ointment on it with a white powder sprinkled over that. When this was all finished they put me into a suit of pajamas instead of the nightshirt I'd been wearing. They picked me up, wrapped a blanket around me, and put me in a big armchair in front of a fire. They placed my feet in a crock half full of hot water and something else that smelled like whiskey. Then they fed me. That was the best meal I ever ate.
>
> There was a large piece of breast meat on the plate. 'Capon!' the widow said. She made motions as if she were lifting something very heavy. Then she blew her chest and thumped it. They all laughed, and I laughed with them.

In Philadelphia, Harriet Ferrel's mother ignored her doctor's advice.

> Dr. Milton White had told my mother she didn't need to feed me anymore, because I was going to die. But you know how mothers are. No mother listens when someone tells her not to feed her child. She does what she has to do for her children, and doesn't listen to anybody else, and that's what my mother did for me.

A train from Seattle eased slowly into the station at Minneapolis. Mary McCarthy's entire family was sick. Her father, Roy, had guarded them against the conductor who had tried to force them off the train. Mary McCarthy later wrote:

> When we arrived in Minneapolis, there were stretchers on the platform, a wheel chair, redcaps, distraught officials.

Six-year-old Mary and her baby brother Kevin were taken to their grandmother's house. Although they did not know it yet, Mary and Kevin were orphans. Their mother, Tess, died four days after arriving in Minneapolis; Roy lived one day longer. For months, no one told Mary and Kevin what had happened to their parents.

> We became aware, even as we woke from our fevers, that everything, including ourselves, was different. I never forgot those weeks in my grandmother's house, loitering in the dark well of the staircase—waiting for Mama to come home from the hospital.

In Washington, D.C., morbidity and mortality statistics were coming in from all over the world. Dr. Victor Vaughan arrived at a frightening conclusion. "If the epidemic continues its mathematical rate of acceleration," Vaughan calculated, "civilization could easily . . . disappear from the face of the Earth."

But it was Spanish influenza, not civilization, which disappeared.

Chapter 8

Reprieve

On November 11, 1918, the city of Boston awoke to the shrill blast of factory whistles, the gong of church bells wildly ringing, and the wail of fire alarms. The ecstatic delirium commenced. The Armistice had ended the war to end all wars. In the nation's capital, President Wilson slowly adjusted his pince-nez and read the terms of the agreement to Congress. In New York's Times Square, women madly kissed anyone in uniform. Chicago's jubilant citizens donned costumes and danced wildly in the streets. The carillon bells of Pittsburgh's churches gaily chimed "Johnny Get Your Gun" and "Over There." For the second time in a week, Philadelphians celebrated. On November 7, rumors of an armistice had sent joyful Philadelphians racing into the streets; on November 11, Philadelphians did it all over again. In San Francisco thirty thousand people paraded through the streets, waving flags, all happy, all dancing, all singing...all wearing masks.

The Armistice ending World War I went into effect on the eleventh hour of the eleventh day of the eleventh month: four years, three months, and five days after the conflict began. John Deleno of New Haven, Connecticut, remembers:

> The firehouses blew their whistles and the factories blew their
> steam whistles and people ran into the streets banging pots and
> pans together. The boys were coming home! We had a big pa-

rade down Grand Street in New Haven and all the military men marched past in their uniforms, their tin hats, and their leggings. Everyone was waving flags, crying and hugging and kissing.

In Goldsboro, North Carolina, Dan Tonkel and his father were awakened long before dawn.

Men were banging on our door, shouting, "Wake up, wake up!" My father and I went downstairs. We found several of his pool buddies who said the Armistice had been signed. They wanted the American flag my father kept draped in the front window of his store. It was a huge flag—maybe six feet wide, eight or ten feet long; my father kept it in the window of his store to show his patriotism. His buddies wanted the flag for a big parade they were organizing. So my father and I went and opened up the store and took down the flag and gave it to the men. A few hours later, the flag was mounted on a pole, leading a big parade through town.

People poured in the streets, forgetting their fears, hugging and kissing. It was a joyous, joyous time. Throngs paraded through Goldsboro.

Even in Philadelphia, a city so shadowed by death, there was rejoicing. Columba Voltz had recovered from the flu. Her parents were convalescing, as was the neighbor who had nursed the family back to health, then fallen sick herself. And on November 11, the gloomy toll of the funeral bells ceased.

The church bells began to ring again so gloriously. I think every church bell in Philadelphia rang that day. It was the most beautiful thing. Hearing the bells, everyone came out of their houses, congregating again, forgetting about the flu, so happy the war was ending. I felt all the joy come back into my life.

Church bells, sirens, wild, spontaneous parades, tin cans tied to the tails of dogs and cats, creating a mad ruckus as pets raced through city streets. All over the world there were shouts, tears, and kisses. In Paris, a weary doughboy pleaded, "What I want is food. I've had nothing but kisses since breakfast." In London, a bus meandered down Regent Street; on its top deck, wounded soldiers beat out "Tipperary" with their artificial legs. Frenzied villagers poured into the streets of Culey, France, shouting "*Vive la France! Vive l'Amerique!*" Private John Lewis Barkley turned to "Jesse" James. "Seems like everyone in town has gone nuts," Barkley said.

The world had much to celebrate. The war over, and, just like that, the pandemic was waning. Mysteriously, swiftly, Spanish influenza was retreating from the world. In many places, the reign of terror lifted suddenly and abruptly. Katherine Anne Porter's fever broke.

> The light came on, and Miss Tanner said, "Hear that? They're celebrating. It's the Armistice. The war is over, my dear."
> Miranda said, "Open the window, please. I smell death in here."

Of course, Spanish influenza did not simply vanish on the eleventh hour of the eleventh day of the eleventh month. However, in a striking coincidence (although coincidence, most agree, is all it is), world-wide morbidity and mortality rates fell off precipitously around the time of the Armistice. Death rates continued to decline throughout the month of November, and the grim statistics of September and October were never again repeated. Flurries of flu did continue through the spring of 1919, substantial in some places, insubstantial in others. These flurries constituted what most epidemiologists consider the "spring wave" of Spanish influenza—the Lady's final act, as it were.

The world-wide pandemic subsided, as it had begun and proliferated, with randomness and caprice. On November 4, flu was waning in Rome, Stockholm, and Copenhagen, but peaking in Pittsburgh, Amsterdam, Edinburgh, and Rio de Janeiro. Misery continued in beleaguered Spain; in Barcelona alone, one hundred thousand remained sick. On November 10, two thousand Britons died; twenty-four hours later, in a stunning reversal of fate, the numbers dropped precipitously.

In New York City, new cases of flu were decreasing by two thousand a day. Dr. Royal Copeland abolished trade and travel restrictions. In December, however, flu rates again began to rise: twenty-one hundred New Yorkers died in December of influenza and related pneumonia. In January 1919, the death rate climbed still higher. On the West Coast, San Francisco reported only fifty new cases of flu during the first week of December. Then (in a pattern similar to New York's), the numbers again began to climb. Health Commissioner Dr. William Hassler cited several culprits: relapses, the sudden influx of returning soldiers, and sheer foolishness, especially the foolishness of San Francisco's women. "Our women who appear on the streets barefoot, or nearly so, with their abbreviated slippers and thin stockings, are simply inviting an attack of flu." But influenza was on the rise all over California—in San Jose, Santa Cruz, Stockton, San Diego, and many other cities. Surgeon General Rupert Blue warned that the epidemic was still very much alive. Vigilance must not be relaxed.

The caprice of Spanish influenza's spring wave was part of an overall pattern of randomness which even now defies simple explanation. Louisville, Kentucky, suffered a severe spring wave of flu, making three "crests": in October 1918, December 1918, and March 1919. Mortality in San Francisco peaked in October and again in January. In general, the American South, Midwest, and Far West experienced severe spring waves of the flu, but there were many exceptions to this rule. Philadelphia and Albany, for instance, suffered only one violent crest, in the fall. Why? To many, the answer seems obvious—some cities were so saturated with influenza that nearly every resident was exposed to the virus. Those who survived the catastrophic autumn possessed immunity to the disease. To a certain extent, that is probably true. But epidemiologists cite numerous exceptions to this rule. Dr. Warren Winklestein, Historical Epidemiologist at the University of California at Berkeley, cautions against drawing any conclusions about the ebb and flow of the 1918 pandemic. Too many factors were at work in 1918 to ever fully appreciate and analyze. Other than death rates (usually credited to pneumonia), no epidemiological data exists. Any explanation of the pandemic's capricious strike and retreat from town to town, house to house is, Winklestein cautions, pure speculation. What appears bewilderingly random will, in all likelihood, always seem so.

Perhaps the single factor whose contribution seems certain is the First World War. The massive wartime mobilization and movement of peoples created a vulnerable, crowded, turbulent population. The plague-infected rats of Europe's Black Death had been replaced by trucks, trains, ships, and crowded trenches which sped influenza on its way and provided a multitude of discrete sanctuaries in which a sneeze, hurling forth its viral minions, could achieve its full power to infect. Still, this does more to explain the pandemic's explosive pattern of onset than its stumbling retreat, and it does nothing to explain the flu's fickle flirtation with some towns and populations and not others. In Montana, for instance, people noticed that butchers and Methodists did not seem to get sick. All over the world, employees of gas works seemed immune. The same was true of workers in cordite and poison-gas factories. British soldiers at the Front seemed far less vulnerable to the microbe than Germans, Americans, or Italians. No wounded soldier ever developed influenza at Oxford's Southern Base Hospital. And while influenza quickly felled staff in German sanitariums, consumptive patients remained bizarrely unaffected.

The mortality rate in Chicago was three times higher than that of Grand Rapids, Michigan, only two hundred miles away and closely linked by road and rail. Waterbury, like most of the state of Connecticut, was devastated; inexplicably, the towns of Darien and Milford escaped the contagion completely. Mortality rates were highest in Pennsylvania, Montana, Maryland, and Colorado, states with diverse demographics, economics, and geography. Why was the death rate ultimately lower in New York than in Boston, Philadelphia, or Washington, D.C.? In fact, Spanish influenza proliferated and vanished of its own accord, in its own inexplicable way. Not surprisingly, policies on mask-wearing seem to have made no difference. Nevertheless, masks (like vaccines) were often considered by the officials who promoted them to have been just the "magic bullet" their city needed.

On November 21, San Francisco "unmasked." Great fanfare accompanied the unveiling. The San Francisco *Chronicle* savored the city's "victory" over the "German-bred" pestilence:

> When the many chaptered epic of San Francisco's share in the world war shall be written, one of the most thrilling episodes will be the story of how gallantly the city of Saint Francis behaved when the black-wings of war-bred pestilence hovered over the city with its death, sorrow, and destitution.

In Philadelphia, many believed Dr. C.Y. White's vaccine had proved the great panacea. Beginning on October 19, 1918, thousands of Philadelphians had been inoculated with White's vaccine. Coincidentally, the epidemic began to wane. Emergency hospitals, like the ward in Susanna Turner's parish, closed. On October 24, the phone plugs were pulled on "Filbert 100." On October 27, church services resumed. On October 28, schools reopened. Dr. Wilmer Krusen declared the epidemic had "ceased to exist officially." The *Philadelphia Inquirer* greeted the lifting of closing orders with a final jab at local authorities: "We have passed through a most dismal period, the gloom of which will be lifted by the reopening of places of amusement. They never should have been closed."

Indeed, as the epidemic waned and the obvious emergency faded, public argument over such issues as closings and mask-wearing became more visible, contentious, and divisive. In this land of eclectic citizenry, private enterprise, free press, and stubborn individualists, protest had always been a cherished American value, in theory, if not always in practice. Catastrophe had dimmed the voices of protest. Not so, as the crisis faded. Or had she? Was the wily plague merely taking a breathe? In Wichita, Kansas, where prowling packs of self-appointed "watchdogs" still ensured the enforcement of closures and quarantine limits, commercial leaders took the city to court, and won. In December, the Supreme Court of the state of Kansas declared Wichita's closures illegal. On December 7, as influenza rates again began to rise in San Francisco, Mayor Rolph made the polite announcement, "The Board of Health feels it necessary to resume the wearing of masks, and I, as Mayor of San Francisco, hereby respectfully ask you to do so immediately." This time, however, San Franciscans ignored the Mayor's request. Ninety percent of San Franciscans shunned the gauze, and mask-slackers, of all persuasions and denominations, loudly voiced their displeasure. Christian Scientists called the mask ordinance "subversive of personal liberty and constitutional rights." Civil libertarians declared, "If the Board of Health can force people to wear masks, then it can force them to submit to inoculation, or any experiment or indignity." The merely sensible voiced what had always seemed obvious: that an ordinance requiring citizens to wear a mask in the open air while allowing them to take it off in crowded restaurants was hopelessly misinformed. Businessmen and restaurateurs worried re-masking would depress holiday buying and spending. The *Chronicle* suggested re-masking would "increase the scare." On December 16, after rowdy public hearings, San Francisco's Board of Supervisors defeated the ordinance. But influenza continued to rise. In the third week of January, 3,500 new cases were reported; 310 San Franciscans died. Once again, the Board of Supervisors tackled the dreaded political hot-potato. Opponents argued re-masking would cause "the stilling of song in the throats of singers" and the incarceration of musicians "as they blow their horns going down the street." But this time, the Supervisors voted to re-mask. Oddly, and quite coincidentally, influenza began to wane. San Franciscans remained a grouchy, cantankerous bunch, however. Hundreds were arrested for mask-slacking and an Anti-Mask League was formed—a raucous group which met for shouting matches between mask "moderates" and mask "extremists." The argument raged until February 1, when San Franciscans were legally permitted to do what they were doing anyway—unveiling.

American society raced back from the edge of a terrifying precipice.

All of a sudden, it was over. A shade lifted. Life returned to normal.

—Bill Sardo

After the parade through Goldsboro, main street just opened up again. It was like you'd flipped a switch. Businesses and theaters opened up again. We went back to school. The farmers started to come back with their wagons of produce, and other vendors showed up within a week or two.

—Dan Tonkel

Bars reopened in Philadelphia; fifty-three people were immediately arrested, drunk and disorderly. Across the nation, picture shows flickered back on, Dorothy Gish in "Battling Jane" and Mary Pickford in "Johanna Enlists." Flo-Flo and her chorus of "Perfect Thirty-Six," who had gamely volunteered in Washington's emergency hospitals, were kicking up their heels in Chicago.

The lively commerce of Anna Milani's street had resumed.

All the children were outside again playing. The fisherman came by with his wagon, selling fresh fish. The pushcart salesman was selling his vegetables. My mother came out—all the mothers came out—buying their fish and vegetables.

In Philadelphia's Rittenhouse Square, Columba Voltz and her friend Katherine were playing Red Rover and Lay Low Sleepy again. They were roller skating on the park's gravel paths, or slipping down the street to watch the blacksmith in his fiery shop.

Everything seemed so marvelous. I knew my uncles would be coming home from army camps; and they hadn't gotten sick. Everyone in our family had recovered from the flu and nobody else I knew was sick. We were all very, very happy. The war was over and the flu was practically gone. Peace and health had returned to the city.

The world had passed through the proverbial shadow of the valley of death. Mustard plasters and bottles of castor oil, camphor and rubbing alcohol were returned to America's medicine cabinets. Garlic necklaces and the pungent asafoetida were discreetly and happily disposed of. Women wore frilly caps to hide hair loss. Flu masks were relegated to cleaning rags.

For many, however, the physical effects of the illness lingered, sometimes for months, sometimes for a lifetime. Convalescence was often painfully slow. Feeble, recovering patients hobbled like invalids, gasping for breath. Some remained stone deaf. Others developed disorders of the heart, lungs, and kidneys. Large numbers of young men developed early Parkinson's disease (chronic trembling paralysis), an illness rarely seen in patients under fifty. The first time Katherine Anne Porter climbed out of bed, she fell and broke her arm. The veins in one leg became swollen; she was told she would never walk again. And often not just the body but the mind remained feeble. Encephalitis (inflammation of the brain) left many lethargic, apathetic, and confused, wanting only to sleep.

Many more were left with immeasurable quotients of grief. Husbands had lost wives. Wives had lost husbands. Thousands of the world's children had been orphaned. Pregnant women had died, taking the unborn with them. Families had been fractured or wiped out completely. For some, the loss was unbearable. In Haslev, Denmark, a physician whose entire family had died went quite mad. Neighbors found him seated in his living room, surrounded by his wife and three children, all propped in chairs, dressed in their Sunday best, all dead. People were marked forever by what they had seen, felt, experienced.

> I keep thinking about it. My brothers and sisters—there are eight of us living now—we talk about the flu, how we were all sick, what we went through. We talk about Harry.
>
> —Anna Milani

After the flu, I was a pretty lonely kid. All my friends had died. These were the friends I had played with for years, gone to school with. When I lost them, my whole world changed. People didn't seem as friendly as before, they didn't visit each other, bring food over, have parties all the time. The neighborhood changed. People changed. Everything changed.

—John Deleno

Mary McCarthy never forgot Seattle in the fall of 1918. She never forgot the fateful train ride east, the illness which claimed her parents. She never forgot her mother Tessa, singing in her loud, husky voice or her handsome father, Roy, hiding Easter eggs among the glorious flora of a Seattle backyard. She always remembered how, in her grandmother's house in Minneapolis, she and her brother had prayed for their parents: "Eternal rest grant unto them, O Lord, and let the perpetual light shine upon them."

For some, the flu revealed a frightening truth about life—and death.

A child never thinks of death. A child thinks he's going to live forever. But I was surrounded by death. I was constantly reminded of the terror and the danger and the finality of death. The flu left an indelible mark on me.

—Bill Sardo

When my mother died, I realized, for the first time and forever, that we are not safe, we are not beyond harm. My father did what he could. He kept us together as a family, but from that time on there was a sadness which had not existed before, a deep down sadness that never went away. We aren't safe. Nobody's safe. Terrible things can happen to anyone at any time.

—William Maxwell

In Denver, Katherine Anne Porter was handed a letter. Her lieutenant had died of influenza. Porter later wrote:

It was one of the most important and terrible things that happened to me. It simply divided my life in two. He was the one person I ever really loved, the one I might have stayed with and been happy with.

Porter's hair grew back. Her arm and leg healed. But 1918 left a wound on her heart which never mended. Many years passed before Porter was able to write "Pale Horse, Pale Rider." The story concludes with sadness, grief, depression, fatigue, the strange and terrible duty of the survivor to carry on, to live.

> No more war, no more plague, only the dazed silence that follows the ceasing of the heavy guns; noiseless houses, empty streets, the dead cold light of tomorrow. Now there would be time for everything.

The Spanish Lady had entered a world of conflict and revolution. She withdrew from a world stage no less dramatic or uncertain.

Germany was in revolt. Sailors and soldiers mutinied, sending red flags flying over Kiel, Hamburg, Bremen, Stuttgart, Munich, and Cologne. Councils of workers and soldiers claimed the power to govern. Knowing Kaiser Wilhelm would never surrender or abdicate, Prince Max of Baden had engineered the Armistice by simply announcing the abdication. Still weak with flu, he stood on the balcony of Berlin's Chancellery, speaking the words the Kaiser would never utter. Two days later, Wilhelm fled across the Dutch border to exile in Holland and Germany's new Chancellor, Social Democrat Friedrich Ebert, authorized the signing of the Armistice. The Russians, too, were embroiled in civil war. The execution of Tsar Nicholas II and his family in the fall of 1918 had made Russia's radical change of course a *fait accompli*. The Communist government of Vladimir Lenin and Leon Trotsky was engaged in bloody civil war with a host of insurgents and counterrevolutionary forces. The vast territory of the old Tzarist empire was in chaos and, to the dismay of many in the West, Bolshevism was winning converts in eastern and central Europe.

In this complex, turbulent world, a critical peace would be decided in Europe. Not quite a year earlier, Woodrow Wilson had addressed the United States Congress, proposing a peace of reconciliation, "a peace without victory," and the establishment of a democratic League of Nation to watch over the world and ensure that the carnage of the Great War would never be repeated. Wilson's decision to continue troop-shipments to Europe despite the devastating pandemic had probably secured the Allied victory. The frail, scholarly Wilson was the undisputed leader of the mightiest nation on Earth. Upon his shoulders rested the burden of reconciling the eternally quarrelsome nations of Europe and convincing the world to act in league for the creation of a world governing body. John Maynard Keynes later wrote, "Never had a philosopher held such weapons wherewith to bind the princes of the world." Peace would be decided in Paris, and the mighty gathered there: Woodrow Wilson; Wilson's chief aide, Colonel Edward M. House; British Prime Minister David Lloyd George; and French Prime Minister Georges Clemenceau. Allies in name, but often at adversarial purpose, they had only one thing in common. Each man had suffered, or would suffer, the sickness and malaise of Spanish influenza. The last to be stricken would be Woodrow Wilson. In this, perhaps her costliest act, the Spanish Lady quite possibly changed the course of twentieth-century history.

Cheering throngs lined the docks of New York. On December 4, 1918, the *George Washington* steamed out of sight of Liberty Island into the vast swells of the Atlantic, carrying its presidential cargo. Woodrow Wilson remarked to an advisor:

Well, Tumulty, this trip will either be the greatest success or the supremest tragedy in all history; but it is my faith that no body of men however they concert their power or their influence can defeat this great world enterprise, which after all is the enterprise of Divine mercy, peace, and good will.

Wilson arrived in Brest, France, to a frenzied ovation. He was welcomed with similar gusto in Paris and Rome. Despite the outpouring of gratitude and joy, few in Europe considered the task of the Paris Peace Conference one of "Divine mercy, peace, and good will." It had been a long, murderous war. One million Frenchmen had died in the trenches of the Western Front; 750,000 Britons had perished. In a speech at the Sorbonne in Paris, Wilson described a "great wind of moral force moving through the world." Undoubtedly, neither Britain's David Lloyd George nor French Prime Minister Clemenceau felt, or could afford to feel, more than a ripple of this warm, Wilsonian breeze. Lloyd George had won re-election in December 1918 with slogans like "Hang the Kaiser"; as reparations, he was demanding nothing less than the complete annexation of Germany's overseas colonies. Clemenceau, too, had promised the French a punishing peace, a peace which would permanently cripple Germany. Privately, he assured his Chamber of Deputies that the Versailles Treaty would be completely devoid of Woodrow Wilson's "noble simplicity."

Paris had endured a long, hard season of sickness and death, and the Spanish Lady was not done with her yet. Brisk flurries of influenza continued throughout the winter (cresting the week of February 22, 1919, when 2,676 Parisians died). Diplomats and aides in all the delegations fell sick. An army physician attending the American delegation complained, "This old world is badly germ-ridden. It is soaked with disease." But even before they reached the Old World, the American delegation had been badly compromised by influenza. In November, the three principal members of the American Peace Commission—Joseph C.

Grew, Walter Lippmann, and Willard Straight—all developed influenza. Straight, described as a man "who could not be spared," died. Then Colonel Edward M. House, Woodrow Wilson's most valued advisor, became sick. House suffered a precarious convalescence and a lingering aftermath of fatigue and malaise. Whether for reasons of health, politics, or both, a rift developed between House, the practical, seasoned tactician, and Wilson, a rift which many historians believe had profound implications for the tragically flawed Treaty of Versailles.

Students of history learn that the seeds of World War II were sown in the punishing, punitive peace of World War I. In fact, the seeds of World War II were sown in a series of cramped rooms in Paris. By March 1919, the Paris Peace Conference had become a discussion among four men. The Big Four, as they were called—the leaders of the United States, Great Britain, France, and Italy, Wilson, George, Clemenceau, and Vittorio Orlando (or, increasingly, the Big Three, minus Italy's Orlando)—would determine the fate of Europe. The men met in Clemenceau's drab office in the Ministry of War, in David Lloyd George's flat, or in the study of Wilson's house on the *Place des Etats-Unis*. Lloyd George later wrote:

> I am doubtful whether any body of men with a difficult task have worked under greater difficulties—stones crackling on the roof and crashing through the windows, and sometimes wild men screaming through the keyholes.

The talks were contentious and hopelessly deadlocked. The devil was not merely in the details, but in the sweeping practical and philosophical meaning of "peace" itself, the questions of German reparations and the (re)drawing of political borders. The world grew impatient. The "Big Four" had become the "Incompetent Four." Europe was in turmoil, hungry and beset with revolution. Germany and Russia remained embroiled in civil war. On

March 22, Hungary fell to the "Reds." American diplomat William C. Bullit told Wilson bluntly, "Six months ago all the peoples of Europe expected you to fulfill their hopes. They believe now that you cannot. They turn, therefore, to Lenin." The pressure upon Wilson to compromise on his "peace of reconciliation" was increasingly coming not just from Europe but from home. In the fall elections, Wilson's Democrats had lost control of both houses of Congress. The stunning Republican victory clearly compromised Wilson's authority abroad. The Chairman of the Senate Foreign Affairs Committee warned the American people against "specious devices of supra-national government" (i.e., Wilson's League of Nations) which could draw the country into the international turmoil. The President knew he lacked the votes in the Senate for ratification of a truly Wilsonian peace. And the public mood was hardly more charitable. Many Americans still blamed the scourge of Spanish influenza on Hun espionage and germs.

In 1913, when Wilson first took office, the distinguished Philadelphia physician, Dr. S. Weir Mitchell, doctor to the mighty and vigorous proponent of the "rest cure" for female hysteria, had predicted that Wilson would not survive his first term. Wilson had defied him. But in the smoky flats of Clemenceau's Paris, he tired. He put off his physician, Dr. Cary T. Grayson, saying, "We are running a race with Bolshevism and the world is on fire. Let us wind up this work here and then we will go home and find time for a little rest."

On the evening of Thursday, April 3, Woodrow Wilson developed a cough. His cough quickly worsened. It became hacking, convulsive, robbing him of breath. He was put to bed. His temperature soared to 103 degrees. Grayson diagnosed influenza. For five days, Wilson languished with symptoms now dreaded the world over. Clemenceau, Lloyd George, and Edward House (appointed by Wilson to take his place in the negotiations) met in the study outside Wilson's sickroom. After House reported a continuing stalemate, "the most footless of many footless meetings," Wilson confided to his wife, "If I have lost the fight, which I would not have done had I been on my feet, I will retire in good order; so we will go home."

Five days after a feeble Wilson rejoined the talks, a deal was struck. Clemenceau yielded, but Wilson yielded more. Wilson's "peace without victory" had become a whole scale condemnation of Germany. When the Treaty of Versailles was completed in May, Wilson told an aide, "If I were a German, I think I should not sign it." Wilson had lost the fight. He had lost, it seemed, the will and stamina to fight.

Many close to him noticed the weakness of both body and mind. Lloyd George later referred to Wilson's "nervous and spiritual breakdown in the middle of the Conference." Herbert Hoover, a close friend, spoke of the difference in Wilson after his illness:

> Prior to that time, in all matters with which I had to deal, he was incisive, quick to grasp essentials, unhesitating in conclusions, and most willing to take advice from men he trusted. After that time, others as well as I found we had to push against an unwilling mind.

Gilbert Close, Wilson's secretary, noted on April 7, "I never knew the President to be in such a difficult frame of mind as he is now. Even while lying in bed he manifested peculiarities." Wilson's left eye and the left side of his face began to twitch. He seemed to many observers, indecisive, forgetful, even paranoid. He wondered if his French servants were spies. When furniture was removed from his apartment, he became agitated, believing he would be held responsible for "acts of thievery."

Students of history wonder why Woodrow Wilson, the uncompromising idealist, compromised. Historian Alfred Crosby suggests:

He who cannot make decisions perforce accepts the decisions of others. Perhaps the most poignant of all the case histories of those who fell ill with Spanish influenza is that of the man who took upon himself the task of ending all wars and lifting humanity to a new level of moral excellence, and whose mind, at one of the crucial moments of modern history, went lame.

Like the lingering flurries of Alaska's long winter, influenza persisted in America's wildest province throughout the spring of 1919. But even before the plague ended, bills were coming due. Alaska's governor, Thomas Riggs, Jr., had spent thousands of dollars bills on relief and medical supplies, quarantine guards, and caring for orphans and convalescents. Burying the dead, a Herculean task in this land of icy snow and frozen earth, had alone cost over $11,000. In January 1919, Alaska's Bureau of Education was feeding hundreds of natives, entirely without the financial means to do so. Governor Riggs declared dejectedly, "I have exceeded my authority in authorizing the care of natives and whites and am, in fact, technically guilty of a criminal offense with a possible jail sentence of six months, but I could not stand by and see our people dying like flies without making an attempt to alter their condition no matter what the consequences." Riggs went to Washington, asking for money, but few in the nation's capital were familiar with the Land of the Northern Lights. The million-dollar appropriation to the Public Health Service had long since been spent. Congress gave him nothing. Riggs wrung $25,000, an eighth of what he needed, from the Red Cross. Discouraged and disillusioned, he returned home and vanished into the wilderness to hunt bears.

Later, in a report to the Federal Secretary of the Interior, Riggs wrote:

I doubt if similar conditions existed anywhere in the world—
the intense cold of the arctic days, the long distances to be
traveled by dog team, the living children huddled against their
dead parents already being gnawed by wolfish dogs.

His bitterness was obvious as Riggs noted the neglect of federal
authorities who were "all too much engrossed with the woes of
Europe to be able to note our wards...dying by swarms in the
dark of the northern nights."

The season of plague was over. Insurance companies, statisti-
cians, leaders of business and industry sharpened their pencils.
What had Spanish influenza cost? Beyond the incalculable—
grief, the loss of human life—were the tallies of government
debt, loss to businesses, and payouts to insurance beneficiaries.
Still, like the immeasurable quotients of heartache and death,
the epidemic's true economic cost remained, and continues to remain, beyond estimation. A hint of these economic costs can be
gleaned from life insurance figures. In the autumn of 1918, even
before the epidemic began to wane, the Metropolitan Life Insurance Company paid out more than $18 million in initial claims
from the beneficiaries of eighty-five thousand life insurance policies. In December 1918, President Henry Moir of the Actuarial
Society of America, a group dedicated to computing insurance
risks and premiums, calculated that because the average flu victim died at age thirty-three, deaths in the nation represented an
economic waste of ten million years. Perhaps more comprehensi-
bly, the city of Philadelphia registered an economic loss of ap-
proximately $60 million. In Kansas, the Spanish Lady's "home
state," the economic loss was calculated at $100 million.

In the winter of 1920, Spanish influenza made its final appear-
ance. In January and February 1920, the nation suffered its high-

est death rate of the century for influenza and pneumonia with the exception of the two preceding years. Outbreaks were most severe in Detroit, Milwaukee, Minneapolis, and St. Louis. The virus continued to show a propensity for the young, but the human population had grown more resistant and the virus had changed. Indeed, the delicate strands of RNA known as Spanish influenza had changed and would continue to change until the virus known as the Spanish Lady simply ceased to exist.

On March 17, 1919, John Lewis Barkley stood rigidly at attention in a parade ground in Andernach, Germany. The field was crowded with divisions of soldiers, blaring military bands, podiums jammed with members of the military brass. John Barkley had long since given up wondering where the mercurial fates of war would lead him and he did not question his purpose in Andernach. He heard his name called. He stepped forward and marched with a group of men towards a flag-draped podium. He glanced up. Barkley had never seen John "Black Jack" Pershing, but he recognized him at once. General Pershing was addressing the crowd, speaking about, "decorating as brave soldiers as the world has ever seen." Barkley listened, rapt. Pershing descended from the podium. He approached Barkley. Barkley automatically snapped a salute. Pershing pumped Barkley's trembling hand and congratulated "a fellow Missourian." No one had ever mentioned Barkley's lone stand at Cunel, that October afternoon spent inside a smoky, bullet-pocked tank, firing round after round at advancing Germans, but Barkley realized he was about to be given a medal. Pershing fumbled with Barkley's shirt. Barkley gasped. The pin had pierced through his blouse, going cleanly into his chest.

Pershing moved away, making his way slowly down the line of men. Barkley looked down and saw a small blue ribbon adorned with stars. He had been pinned with the Congressional Medal of Honor—the highest award an American soldier could attain.

On the edge of a ruddy canyon outside Meadow, Utah, the Pahvant Indians took down their tents and moved away. Lee Reay recalls, "They were afraid and they just left. I don't know where they went."

The Evangelical preachers returned to Harriet Ferrel's neighborhood in Philadelphia.

> This time, the people listened. The ministers' prophecy had been fulfilled. Listening to them, people had a kind of religious awakening. It could have been fear. Fear can be good, it can sometimes make you do the right thing, make you turn to God. I don't know what causes illness and calamities and tumults, but there's a God who looks down on the universe; he's the creator and the sustainer of man—and sometime man gets so clever and thinks he doesn't need a power above himself. We bring a lot of calamities on ourselves, because we're so hotheaded and stubborn. I think the plague happened for a reason.

Selma Epp's mother visited the Philadelphia Board of Health. Her son Daniel had died of influenza. He had been taken away in a corpse-filled cart, as required by emergency city ordinance. Selma recalls:

> The people at the Philadelphia Health Department said they didn't know where Daniel was buried. He had been buried somewhere in a mass grave; they didn't know where. My mother had been too weak with protest when Daniel was taken away and she never forgave herself. Daniel was her first-born son. That he had been buried in a mass grave, that

she never knew where, that she could not visit his grave, light a candle for his death was so painful to her that she was never able to talk about it. Whenever the subject was mentioned, her eyes filled with tears.

In October 1918, "a girl" was buried in a mass grave too, in the "Trench" of Holy Cross cemetery. "A Polish man and his baby" were buried in each other's arms in a plain wooden box. Neither the girl nor the Polish man and his baby were known to the family of Michael Donohue, who buried them. Perhaps a mother, a father, or a sister like Selma Epp mourned them. Perhaps not. Perhaps the sister, the mother, the father had already died of influenza. Selma Epp's mother never forgave herself for allowing her son to be buried in a mass grave. But for Michael Donohue, Philadelphia's "trenches," the most inhumane of grave sites, represented an act of bold, vigorous humanity and charity. It was simply the only way to get things done.

The truth is that even at the height of the chaos, America never quite fell apart. In the fall of 1918, many locked their doors and stayed inside. Some abandoned their sick relatives or, lacking means or strength, left bodies in alleys. But many more ventured out to help—to nurse the sick and to bury the dead. In many places, "hospitals" were hopelessly crude, but hospitals they were. In most hospitals, nurses were not nurses, but they nevertheless nursed the sick. Whether bedded down in a school, a musty library, or a tent pitched on Boston's muddy Corey Hill, flu victims received care by people whose courage is impossible to overestimate. Despite the lack of a medical infrastructure—a pervasive and powerful Public Health Service, a sophisticated network of hospitals, health professionals, and medical researchers, and scientists capable of providing therapeutic relief—communities conspired, in a myriad of curious, inventive ways, to provide the sip of water, the warm blanket, the clean sheet, and ultimately, when that failed, the burial shroud and, when available, the coffin.

Perhaps in some respects the America of 1918 was better prepared for such a tragedy than we might be today. Today, we deposit our sick in hospitals and fill their rooms with cards and flowers. In 1918, a family bedroom was often the only hospital most people ever saw, and a mother, sister, or daughter the only nurse. William Maxwell and his brother were cared for by their aunt and uncle—dour, unwelcoming people, but nevertheless "people you could count on in trouble." When family members were unavailable or unwilling, neighbors pitched in. In Philadelphia, Columba Voltz's aunt, the mother of two small sons, did not dare visit the Voltz's sickhouse, but a neighbor did—a woman from the third floor who nursed Columba's parents, then Columba, then fell sick herself. Lee Reay and the other residents of Meadow, Utah, masked themselves like bandits and kept their distance, but kept things going. Food was left on doorsteps, cows were milked, pigs were fed. Men from Meadow helped Indians at the nearby camp bury their dead.

> We learned a few things in our town during this epidemic. One was that we had an obligation to look after each other. My dad, William H. Reay, covered the whole town every day on his horse, checking to see who was sick, what people needed. It didn't matter whether you were relatives or not, we were one big family in Meadow.

The autumn of 1918 was a nightmarish time. But many would remember the indefatigable courage, the generosity, the goodness of friend and stranger alike. In Macon, Georgia, Katherine Guyler and her mother were desperately sick; Katherine's frantic father went out one night in search of a nurse. He searched and searched until he found one at a dance in a neighbor's barn.

My father came home with a woman in a beautiful evening dress. She moved into our house, and nursed us through our long, painful illness.

Can we imagine such a thing happening today?

I have enormous memories of good, good people—people who were hurt, who died, or people who helped each other, sharing in each other's lives. We didn't know then what was ahead for us in this century. I suppose we still don't know what's ahead for us, for America. So much has changed. Nineteen-eighteen was a good good time, a good world.

—Katherine Guyler

Chapter 9

Forgetting

As soon as the dying stopped, the forgetting began. In the end, the epidemic would vanish from our collective memory. Histories of the United States and the world seldom mention the greatest killer we ever had. The medieval Black Death, six hundred years remote, continues to fascinate and horrify, pique our imagination, but the autumn of 1918 was the deadliest season of plague ever. Yet it is the horror story no one remembers.

In history, we read about times when plagues killed so many people, but we never read about what happened to us. Everyone knows about the plague in Europe. I don't know why our plague isn't remembered. It doesn't seem right. People should know. It was a very great trial for us. People who lived through that fall never forgot. I didn't. I never forgot.

—Susanna Turner

I'm an avid reader and I never read anything about the 1918 flu. I'm eighty-five years old and to this day, I still have no idea how far it spread, how many people died. All I know is what happened in my neighborhood in New Haven, Connecticut. I don't know what happened in New York or New Jersey or Vermont. I never heard.

—John Deleno

In four years, the Civil War cost 498,000 lives. In World Wars I and II and the Korean and Vietnam Wars, an estimated 423,000 Americans perished. The Civil War is a national obsession; the horrible, riveting glamour of World War II and the divisive quagmire of Vietnam explode from the pages of history. We visit Gettysburg, reenact Civil War battles. We recall the anniversary of Pearl Harbor, D-Day, and Hiroshima. We run our hands across the granite names on the Vietnam memorial as if blindly probing the faces of the dead.

In ten months, 675,000 Americans died of Spanish influenza.

Why does memory fail us?

The influenza epidemic of 1918 had no William Tecumseh Sherman, no Abraham Lincoln, no Sitting Bull, George Patton, John F. Kennedy, or Ho Chi Minh. In 1918, women and men bravely nursed the sick, putting themselves at grave risk, but theirs was a private battlefield and their foe the most ghostly of enemies. In an explosive convulsion of epidemic disease, Spanish influenza attacked twenty-five million Americans. She took more American lives than the twentieth century's greatest villain, Adolf Hitler. But this invisible killer could not make us, in our engagement with her, glorious.

In 1918, such paradoxical logic was not lost on America's military commanders. Doughboys felled by Spanish influenza or by wounds sustained in battle were, in the end, all remembered as casualties of war. Morale and the human heart demanded nothing less. The pride of a soldier is his strength, his muscle and will. How much better to die a soldier's death than to succumb to the "flu": a common, household disease. In the fall of 1918, 621,000 American servicemen fell sick with influenza, reduced in a matter of hours to prone, delirious invalids—hardly a boost for morale or fodder for legend. Despair over the physical collapse of soldiers was obvious in the final report of the Navy's chief medical officer. Most who died, he lamented, "were robust young men when attacked, and the number of these well-developed and well-nourished bodies at necropsy made a spectacle sad beyond description." No one understood the demands of morale better than Army Chief of Staff General Payton March. Calling for the continuation of troop shipments to Europe despite the obvious peril of plague, March had insisted that every doughboy who died of influenza on an Atlantic troopship, "has just as surely played his part as his comrade who has died in France." Similarly, at memorial services for influenza victims in Camp Meade, Maryland, the reading of a soldier's name was followed by the snap of his Sergeant's salute and the terse explanation, "Died on the field of honor, sir." For forty-three thousand American doughboys, the "field of honor" was a weirdly civilian place: the cold stone floor of a makeshift hospital, the heaving deck of a troopship, or a dilapidated porch in the middle of the Kansas badlands, pelted by rain. And for families mourning the loss of a son, the cause of death must have seemed less important than knowing he died a soldier among soldiers, engaged in the grand enterprise of war.

Innocence is the stuff of childhood. Nineteen-eighteen was a complex moment in history. Nineteen-eighteen was a year not simply of global altercation, but of conflict and ambivalence within the hearts of nations and the hearts of individuals. Patriotic Americans led Liberty Loan Drives. Schoolchildren saved their pennies for Thrift stamps. Francis Russell and the children of Dorchester baked peach pits for a befuddling, if shining purpose. Germans were denounced as "vile Huns" and effigies of Kaiser Wilhelm went up in flames across the nation. Other Americans—like the century's first "draft-dodgers," unconvinced of an American obligation to "Martyred Belgium," like Katherine Anne Porter, who recoiled at the coercive techniques of Liberty Bond salesmen and appeals like "Give till it hurts," like some residents of Macon, Georgia, who quietly debated the sudden influx of strangers into their heartland—were unpersuaded of a clear moral imperative in the European war.

On November 11, 1918, the Armistice was signed and the Spanish Lady began her swift, sporadic retreat. Truly, she had not stayed long. It was precisely the terrifying swiftness with which she engulfed Earth which led to her sudden demise. Serum antibody levels later revealed that nearly every person alive in 1918 had been exposed to the virus. Global infection produced global immunity. As medical historian Dr. Sheila Fannin asserts, "Like a firestorm, the pandemic swept across the world. Then, like a fire without fuel, it was gone." Perhaps the transient swiftness of the pandemic contributed to the world's amnesia.

In a single month, 12,162 Philadelphians perished.

Influenza claimed 85 percent of the population of Teller Mission (now Brevig Mission), Alaska.

In Kansas, 174,094 became sick. Twelve thousand died.

In the closing week of October 1918, 2,700 Americans soldiers died on the battlefields of Europe. That week, 21,000 Americans died at home of Spanish influenza.

Once the trauma had passed, wasn't it better to forget? Francis Russell later wrote:

> By November the influenza had passed, and in the turbulence of the war's ending it tended to be forgotten quickly. So many had died since 1914, but it was over now, all the killing and the dying, and better to start again and put death out of mind. For all its deaths, influenza did not last long enough to stamp itself permanently on the popular imagination. And in any case, like the war, it was part of the past. The present was what mattered.

Experience is gained at a price. The price is often a loss of innocence, and most of us relinquish innocence only with the greatest reluctance, a little bit at a time, assisted by of those eternal helpmates of the human heart: denial, self-deception, feelings of invincibility ("it will never happen again"), the distortions of memory, and the dreamy inventions of nostalgia. Perhaps we have forgotten the pandemic because, in a way, we never knew about it. No nation on Earth spoke insistently and openly about the carnage. Many American officials like Rupert Blue, Louis Brownlow, William Hassler, Samuel Crumbine, and Senator John Weeks fought the good fight. But many more denied the threat, procrastinated, and waffled. Many, following the lead of the President himself, continued to prioritize Liberty Loan rallies, parades, and "patriotic sings," despite the obvious threat to the public health. In November 1918, even as influenza was killing five thousand New Yorkers a week, the *New York Times* observed, "Perhaps the most notable peculiarity of the influenza epidemic is the fact that it has been attended by no traces of panic or even of excitement." In *The Plague of the Spanish Lady*, historian Richard Collier muses:

> Even at the height of the slaughter, there was this same ambivalence. The disease took at least half a million American lives ... yet only in the hardest-hit cities did it ever win through to the newspapers' front pages.... To some medical men, at least, the fate of civilization hung in the balance, for medicine could do little more than in the Middle Ages, when a red cross painted on the door of a stricken house, with the legend "God have pity on us," was the sum total of medical knowledge. Yet no such stark facts were ever voiced by the world's headlines.

Historian A. A. Hoehling agrees. "There was, apparently, a tacit conspiracy among the nation's editors to hush-hush the ever-mounting ravages, as though they hoped that if they did not notice, the infection would go away." The same was true all over the world. In Zurich, Switzerland, the Director of Public Health appealed to the editors of the city's newspapers: "Please don't mention influenza in your obituary notices." In New Zealand, the government steadfastly refused to reveal morbidity and mortality statistics. In many nations, bureaucratic silence became justified by wartime censorship. Denial was considered essential to a nation's security. Silence was institutionalized.

By conservative estimate, 450,000 Russians died of Spanish influenza, 375,000 Italians perished, 228,000 Britons, and 225,000 Germans.

In October 1918, India suffered a month of disease unparalleled in the history of human civilization. Between twelve and twenty million people died on the Indian subcontinent.

Given the catastrophe, perhaps the loudest silence of all came from the world's most powerful leader, Woodrow Wilson. In September 1918, Wilson spoke out in favor of suffrage for women. On October 12, he led a throng of twenty-five thousand flag-waving patriots through the streets of flu-ridden New York. Throughout the fall, in a daring philosophical gamble, Wilson continued to proselytize about a world governing body, even as Earth's population was being felled by the millions. Wilson made no such speeches and led no such drives against Spanish influenza. He made no attempt to mobilize national or global consciousness to fight the microbe's legions. Wilson was busy fighting a war with visible enemies. It did not take a medical man to know that in his contest with the pandemic, man's weapons were hopelessly crude. In the war against Spanish influenza, men were profoundly, disturbingly impotent.

In four years, three months, and five days, World War I claimed some ten million lives. In ten months, Spanish influenza killed between twenty-one and forty million people.

It was horrible. It's no wonder we never talked about it. No wonder that people who lived through it just wanted to forget, to move on, just move on. It's no wonder. No wonder.

—Michael Donohue

On the one-year anniversary of my mother's death, my mother's sister threw a party. It was an odd thing to do. I still don't understand it, but people grieve in their own strange ways. All the friends of our family came, including their children. My father filled the house with red roses and for the first time since my mother died I had a good time. I played with the other children and it was lovely, it was happy, it was the way it used to be. I didn't realize what the occasion was until I heard one of my aunts say, "Will [Maxwell's father] is very quiet tonight," and then I realized it was the anniversary of my mother's death. I was ashamed that I had been happy. I should have been grieving.

—William Maxwell

In all likelihood, the twin tragedies of war and Spanish influenza visited trauma upon every household in America. What could be more devastating than bearing witness to mass death? What could be more painful than to watch mothers, fathers, siblings, and children die? In the fall of 1918, friendly neighbors vanished behind locked doors and were carried out as corpses. "Death carts" rattled down deserted city streets. Morgues and graveyards overflowed. To some at least, the "death" of human civilization seemed imminent. Historian Alfred Crosby suggests America came too close to social breakdown to be able to "remember." He titles a final chapter in his definitive history of the pandemic, *Epidemic and Peace, 1918*, "An Inquiry into the Peculiarities of Human Memory." Perhaps, Crosby speculates, we have forgotten what we cannot bear to know. During that deadly October, America seemed poised on the brink of chaos. Modern medicine, with nothing to offer, fell victim to superstition. Man's "higher emotions" became casualties of fear. Many fled into a place of profound alienation even from family, a place ruled by a basic instinct to survive, to save oneself.

> I don't know why, but everything was forgotten. The flu was forgotten as far as people were concerned.
>
> —Columba Voltz

> I wonder why the flu did not impress people more than it did, the loss of millions of human lives. As soon as the disease subsided, everyone just went back to their normal way of living. They grieved, of course; but once the fact became embedded in them that their loved ones were gone, they put it behind them and tried to carry on with their lives. People blocked it out of their minds, the way people block out terrible events. People just don't want to remember how horrible it was.
>
> —Dan Tonkel

Had the pandemic not occurred during a season of war, would it have impressed us more, then and now? Perhaps. History, recorded by humans, is not immune to the exigencies of the human heart. In *The Pursuit of Liberty: A History of the American People*, R. Jackson Wilson et. al. write, "To some extent, the practice of ignoring, evading, or denying reality is a characteristic of culture in any society." The collective memory of a nation, a people, a race, or a tribe often becomes subject to the wishes, distortions, and denials which make individual memory so fallible a vessel for objective truth. In 1918, families, neighborhoods, cities, nations, and the world itself moved through the same stages of bewilderment, denial, engagement, and horror as individuals did. Forgetting was no exception. Perhaps the global amnesia attending Spanish influenza is less the result of distraction by war than because the tragic lessons of World War I were so hard to bear. The first bloody war in mankind's bloodiest century, World War I is widely regarded as the war in which war lost its "romance." The machinery of modern warfare wrought savage, unprecedented, profoundly impersonal devastation. There was hardly an echo of the daring cavalry charge in doughboys scrambling from nightmarish trenches into "no man's land," to be killed in a matter of seconds. At the end of the war, hundreds of thousands of soldiers returned home, suffering from an illness which bore eerie resemblance to nineteenth-century female hysteria. Shell shock, as it came to be known, became recognized as physical and emotional debilitation resulting from severe mental trauma. For many, World War I would be remembered as a war without an obvious or explicable cause. Villains and heroes, fading into obscurity, became as unmemorable as the Prussian duke whose assassination had somehow demanded the death of ten million souls. World War I was a pivotal moment in history, a moment in which man simultaneously reveled in and despaired over what he had wrought. The industrial age had created stunning progress—but progress itself had caused the massive scope of the carnage. We called it the war to end all wars, but twenty-seven years later, the Enola Gay whispered through the clouds; Hiroshima's urban grid dissolved in a blinding flash and a rush of greenish wind, ushering in the profound moral tragedy of the Nuclear Age. Perhaps the first whisper of this greenish wind could be heard in the thunder of "Big Bertha" or in the frenzied burst of a Maxim machine gun. Compared to this, the pandemic— without heroes and villains, entirely beyond the reach of man's genius—did not stand a chance.

When I was a very small child, I was riding around with my father in our 1936 Reo. I was sitting in the back seat on a drab olive blanket—a thick, heavy blanket unlike any other blankets we owned. I asked my father where it came from and he said he'd taken it off the cot of someone who died in Camp Devens. Decades later, I was sitting in a library with a complete set of World Almanacs spread out before me. I was looking at mortality rate tables for this century. Everything got better and better in the United States, except in 1918. In 1918, the death rate shot up by about a quarter. I wondered why and I remembered my father and his blanket in the Reo.

I don't think we'll ever understand why we forgot the 1918 pandemic. True, it was overshadowed by war, and wars are heroic and wars are tragic, but the scope of the carnage from Spanish influenza was horrendous. My theory is that God challenged himself to kill as many people as he could without the human species noticing and he came up with influenza— the unimportant disease that you don't have to worry about, that killed millions of people eighty years ago. As long as we breathe, we risk getting influenza. It would be the worst, the silliest kind of optimism to say, "It happened once, it will never happen again." Yes it will.

—Alfred Crosby, historian

Despite the bitter lessons of World War I, the Allied triumph brought glory, pride, and a sense of powerful mastery to the victors. Influenza was a riddle within a puzzle within a mystery, a cryptic conundrum which science could neither decipher, understand, or control. Spanish influenza waxed and waned according to her own inscrutable logic. Science was powerless at the beginning and powerless at the end. Medical men did not defeat her— she simply withdrew: millions of microscopic legions retreating without surrender—even, in the end, in defiance of science. Dr. Kenneth F. Maxcy of the U.S. Public Health Service called Spanish influenza "an appalling demonstration of man's helplessness and ignorance." Dr. Victor Vaughan later recalled:

The saddest part of my life was when I witnessed the hundreds of deaths of the soldiers in the Army camps and did not know what to do. At that moment I decided never again to prate about the great achievements of medical science and to humbly admit our dense ignorance in this case. There can be no armistice between medicine and disease. The conflict will continue as long as man walks the earth and the victory will ultimately be won by death.

Science could not forget. Science had failed utterly. And so science went in search of ever-smaller mysteries, the faceless, Lilliputian microbe which had obliterated millions.

All over the world, medical researchers intensified their work. The tools of bacteriology were refined. Techniques used to culture cells (to grow cells in labs and infect them with microbes) became more sophisticated. Increasingly-powerful microscopes yielded ever-smaller secrets. In the decade following the 1918 pandemic, four thousand books and articles were published on influenza. Slowly, painstakingly, bacteriologists invented the field of virology. "Filterable agents" were no longer the subject of speculation. The existence of viruses was now certain. But how do you to catch fireflies with a butterfly net? How do you trap air in your hand?

And so to pigs.

In the autumn of 1918, Iowa's pig farmers had become alarmed. Pigs were big business in Iowa; no state in the Union boasted more pigs than Iowa. But at the National Swine Breeders' Show in Cedar Rapids, pigs were falling sick, felled by a savage illness whose high fevers and hacking coughs bore eerie resemblance to the human plague. Rumors circulated that hogs were giving the disease to farmers and vice versa. Pig farmers and medical men alike speculated about a connection. Hundreds of feverish swine were paraded, judged, pinned with or denied ribbons, languishing or dying at the Fair or later, when they returned home. Dr. J. S. Koen, an inspector in the Bureau of Animal Industry's Hog Cholera Control Division, aroused the ire of farmers and meat packers (who feared a loss of consumer confidence in bacon) when he documented the outbreak in *The American Journal of Veterinary Medicine*. Koen stated, "It looked like 'flu,' it presented the identical symptoms of 'flu,' it terminated like 'flu,' and until proved it was not 'flu,' I shall stand by that diagnosis."

Iowa's hogs were not the only ones affected. Sick pigs caused the cancellation of Hagerstown, Maryland's 1918 fair as well. Never before had such an illness been noticed in pigs, but from then on, every fall "swine flu" struck America's hogs.

In 1928, Dr. Richard Shope, a researcher at the Rockefeller Institute's Animal Pathology Lab, set out to explore a possible connection between swine flu and Spanish influenza. Perhaps swine flu would provide clues to human influenza and that elusive, yet-unseen creature, a virus. Scientists were not sure animals could even *get* the flu. Nevertheless, other researchers had the same idea as Shope: find an animal with a flu-like disease, expose the secrets of that disease, and unlock the mysteries of human influenza. Dogs, specifically dogs suffering canine distemper, became the focus of researchers in Boston, New York, and London. Clinically similar to influenza, canine distemper incapacitates dogs with high fevers and weepy eyes and noses, and sometimes proves fatal. In 1921, Britain's Medical Research Council appealed for research dollars from dog and fox-hunting enthusiasts. Within a decade, dog lovers in England and the United States had given the National Institute for Medical Research Farm Laboratories at Mill Hill, England, its budget. Five years later, the virus responsible for canine distemper was isolated; by 1929, a vaccine was in commercial production.

In the fall of 1928, Dr. Richard Shope arrived in Iowa and

found "sick pigs all over the place." Ever since 1918, swine flu had been an autumn ritual in the Midwest, as predictable as the changing of the leaves and the harvesting of the Halloween pumpkin. The conundrum defied explanation. Herds of pigs hundreds of miles apart would fall simultaneously sick. Three months later, the plague would simply vanish. In 1930, Shope isolated the virus responsible for swine flu. In so doing, he became the first scientist to isolate a mammalian influenza virus.

This triumph ensured Shope's immortalization in the annals of science. But Shope was not finished with pigs. For twenty years, he pondered the puzzle of swine flu, and formulated a subtle and ingenious theory to explain its mysterious annual cycles. Shope hypothesized a deadly, synergistic relationship between bacterial and viral agents—Pfeiffer's bacillus and a swine version of the 1918 Spanish flu. He further suggested the import of a parasite, swine lungworm, which inhabits the lungs of pigs and which, according to Shope, acts as a "host cell" in which the flu virus lies dormant (riding the lungworm through its parasitic cycles) until a seasonal combination of Pfeiffer's bacteria and cold, wet, autumn weather causes it to explode to life. Although Scope's theory of a symbiotic relationship between bacterial and viral agents was disproved by later research, his painstaking attention to the most subtle acts of parasitic and microbial behavior and to the bedeviling complexity of the natural world testifies to the difficulty of the challenge. Viruses have proven infinitely more sly and perfidious than the bacteria which revealed themselves to Koch, Pasteur, and other nineteenth-century microbiologists.

What of human influenza? Another animal proved the unwitting hero in the isolation of the human influenza virus: the ferret. An ornery, weasel-like rodent, the ferret came to the attention of researchers at the National Institute for Medical Research Farm Laboratories at Mill Hill, England, the same team which had isolated the virus responsible for canine distemper. In 1933, an influenza epidemic broke out in England. Doctors Wilson Smith, Christopher H. Andrewes, and Patrick P. ("P. P.") Laidlaw swabbed the throats of flu victims and tried to infect laboratory animals with the residue. Like so many others, they failed—until they tried the ferret. Two ferrets were inoculated with influenza "filtrate." On February 4, 1933, Professor Wilson Smith made the droll, triumphant announcement: "Ferret Number One looks somewhat seedy." Indeed, the ferret was sick. Smith's luck continued. The sniffily ferret sneezed in Smith's face. To his immense delight, Smith came down with the flu. The Smith-Andrewes-Laidlaw team had isolated the first human influenza virus. It was named "WS," after the professor upon whom Lady Luck had sneezed.

In the 1960s, the influenza virus was glimpsed for the first time, seen through the powerful lens of an electron microscope. Hardly pernicious or sinister-looking, it is a fluffy, cloud-like creature. Some twelve million influenza viruses can fit on the head of a pin.

A brief aside. What of that notorious distraction, Pfeiffer's bacillus? It was later proven that, although Pfeiffer's bacillus is a frequent invader of cells and tissues, it does not *cause* any specific disease. In 1918, much time was wasted on Pfeiffer's bacillus, but it later led one medical researcher to a critical medical discovery. Pfeiffer's bacillus is a temperamental bacteria, notoriously difficult to grow in a laboratory. It simply will not grow unless cultured in heated blood, in a solution known as chocolate agar. Other bacteria, especially the "cocci": streptococcus, pneumococcus, and others, often overwhelm it, retarding its growth. Dr. Alexander Fleming, a British bacteriologist, returned from service in World War I determined to find a way to prevent the infection of wounds. He also resolved to find the microbe responsible for influenza. For his second purpose, he needed to find a way to inhibit the "cocci" which interfere with the growth of Pfeiffer's *Haemophilus influenzae*. One day, quite by accident, Fleming left several Petri dishes of staphylococci unattended, open to contamination. A natural interloper visited the plates, devouring all the "cocci"—a mold called penicillium.

The "peculiarities" of human memory did not prevent influenza research from progressing, nor did they allow public health officials to ignore the epidemic's hard lesson. Public hygiene was no longer simply the *cause célèbre* of "sanitarians," but mandated by law. States drafted new sanitary codes. Inspections ensured that employees in public establishments like restaurants, hotels, and drugstores wash dishes in scalding hot water, maintain sterile toilets, and perform a host of other small but critical tasks to maintain basic standards of cleanliness. Nineteen-eighteen had been a catastrophe of public health. In its wake, Surgeon General Rupert Blue called for expanded powers and centralization of the U.S. Public Health Service. Other countries heeded the pandemic's message as well. Across the world, in South Africa, France, Australia, Russia, and India, national health departments were created or reinforced. In January 1920, the League of Nations Health Organization (today's World Health Organization) established an international network to coordinate influenza detection and response.

Every day, clinicians all over the swab the runny noses and sore throats of flu sufferers. Specimens are analyzed, and any virus which seems worrisome is sent to a World Health Organization lab—the Centers for Disease Control in Atlanta or laboratories in Melbourne, London, or Tokyo. New strains of influenza are constantly being born as viruses change and mutate, "drift, " and "shift." Viral drift (when a genetic mutation provokes a change in the protein hemagglutinin) renders a previous year's vaccine ineffective. When hemagglutinin (HA) and neuraminidase (NA), the two proteins which encase a virus' core RNA, combine in a completely new way, a virus is said to have "shifted." As viruses drift and shift, they create generation after generation of "offspring." For any virus forwarded to a W.H.O. lab, a complete family tree is constructed. In this way, scientists keep their finger on the microbe's mutable pulse. Since the 1970s, all the strains of influenza circulating through the world's human population have fallen into one of two viral families: H1N1 or H3N2. A virus which falls outside these families will sound an international alarm, because a shift to a new viral family represents a dangerous threat to the human immune system and possesses the potential for a global pandemic. Scientists now believe the 1918 pandemic was the result of a shift to the H1N1 family of viruses. Where did Spanish influenza "go"? Most probably, the virus drifted over the course of forty years, causing occasional outbreaks (in 1947, for instance). In 1957, another shift occurred. The H1N1 family of viruses was replaced by H2N2: the "Asian flu" killed seventy thousand Americans. In 1968, the Hong Kong flu represented yet another shift; twenty-eight thousand Americans died.

The question is not *if* another deadly shift will occur, but *when*. Cyclical seasons of (potential) pandemic are just as inevitable today as in times past, as certain now as during the reign of Justinian or medieval times. Decades lacking a pandemic are referred to as an "inter-pandemic period." Antibiotics can now better control the secondary bacterial infections which often prove fatal in cases of influenza, such as bacterial pneumonia. But in 1918, millions died a swift, terrifying death of *viral* pneumonia. Human beings remain profoundly vulnerable to influenza, especially to strains which represent an interspecies' combination of viruses—a duck-pig-human virus, for example. The World Health Organization, therefore, lavishes special attention upon regions of the world where waterfowl, pigs, humans, and domestic poultry live in close proximity to one another. China, for instance. There, the mingling and recombination of viruses within animal "mixing vessels" such as pigs invites the creation of dangerous hybrid viruses which are most threatening to man.

Every winter, the United States Food and Drug Administration hosts an annual "Flu Meeting." Public health officials, scientists, and pharmaceutical manufacturers gather to form an educated guess about what influenza virus will most likely dominate the following autumn. It takes up to six months to manufacture a vaccine, so pharmaceutical companies must know by February or March what virus to target in order to spare the world's population the annual misery of the flu. At the Flu Meeting, the Centers for Disease Control presents a detailed map of world-wide viral activity. Keeping close tabs on genetic mutations helps scientists predict which strains will most likely prove dominant. In the past, these predictions were notoriously off target. Since the 1980s, the guesses have been near-perfect.

Nevertheless, an outbreak of so-called "bird flu" in Hong Kong in August 1997 revealed just how much remains beyond the reach of science. In August 1997, influenza appeared in Hong Kong. It seemed to be spread by chickens; a million chickens were slaughtered. Between August and December 1997, the Hong Kong "bird flu" infected eighteen people and killed six. Such an outbreak might seem statistically unremarkable, except for one alarming fact. Until this, scientists had never documented an incident in which birds transmitted influenza *directly* to human beings. Influenza viruses originate and exist naturally (and usually harmlessly) in birds, but it was believed that a "bridge species" (pigs, for instance) was necessary in order to introduce influenza to the human population. Have birds *always* been able to transmit influenza directly to human beings? In 1997, did scientists simply "catch" what has always been happening? Can a completely avian virus (a bird flu) become established in people, spread *effectively* from human to human, and develop into a pandemic strain? Or are avian viruses simply becoming ever-more-ingenious, more capable of infecting and compromising people?

The 1997 Hong Kong "bird flu" demonstrates just how much remains beyond the scope of twentieth-century science, and offers yet more testimony of the wily, adaptive genius of viruses.

In Royal Copeland's New York City, 33,387 people died of Spanish influenza. Still, numbers are little help in calculating human loss. Ultimately, experience is not about the dead or the sheer number of dead, but about the living, those who remember, forget, or, through the circuitous channels of memory, half-live and half-die with the loss. Each human death resonates against the living, creating currents of grief, acceptance, bitterness, and wisdom which—like the proverbial pebble tossed into a pond—continue to ripple long after the initial pain has subsided and long after conscious memory fails.

Michael Wind grew up in Brooklyn, New York.

> The age span for people like myself is running out. The people of my generation are fast disappearing. Nevertheless, there is still time to tell the story...
>
> In 1918, I was a six-year-old youngster watching firemen race down the street, horses galloping, their nostrils flaring...
>
> When the influenza epidemic hit, children my age didn't understand what was happening. History was being made, but all we knew was that people were dying and we'd help by standing in front of a deceased person's house, collecting coins for the funeral.

Michael's mother died of influenza. Michael and his five brothers and sisters were gathered together. Michael's father was weeping.

Looking at my mother, I could not relate to my loss. She looked like she was asleep.

The next morning, their father bought Michael and his two younger brothers a Hershey bar. Then he placed them in the Brooklyn Hebrew Orphan Asylum.

Michael Wind grew up. He married. He and his wife Luna raised a daughter. Luna was diagnosed with Alzheimer's disease; she died in 1995. Devastated, Michael sought help in an Alzheimer's support group. Then, at age eighty-four, he entered therapy. He could not rid himself of his depression and grief, until one day when his therapist said simply, "She was not your mother. Your wife was not your mother."

It was like living in a dark room for all these years and a door was opened and a ray of daylight came through. Ever since that day I saw my mother lying on the bed, my father sobbing uncontrollably, I had been searching for her. I was happy at the Hebrew Orphan Asylum; I never knew—I never guessed how much I was grieving. The therapist's words, that my wife Luna had not been my mother, made it all clear to me. That was the last session I had with my therapist. I had my answer.

My saga began the day I entered the Hebrew Orphan Asylum at age six and ended with my last analysis session at age eighty-six. All my life, I had been unconsciously seeking my mother, without realizing it. It has been a long road to travel, but now I understand. Thoughts do not come easy at eighty-seven. But as of today, everything is holding and in place.

Epilogue

In July 1996, Dr. Amy Krafft, one of a team of molecular biologists at the Armed Forces Institute of Pathology in Washington, D.C., took a razor blade and carefully shaved a fleck of lung tissue loose from a minute paraffin block. The scrap of preserved lung had belonged to a twenty-one-year-old Army private, Private Roscoe Vaughn. On September 19, 1918, Private Vaughn fell sick with Spanish influenza. He died on September 26, 1918, at 6:30 A.M., of massive pneumonia at Fort Jackson, South Carolina. At 2 P.M., an autopsy was performed. A pathologic specimen was sliced from his lung, soaked in formaldehyde, preserved in a small chunk of paraffin wax (about a half-inch in diameter), and sent to Washington, D.C. For nearly eighty years, the minuscule fragment of Private Vaughn's lung remained discretely housed in the vast reaches of the National Tissue Repository. A massive U.S. Army pathologic warehouse, the National Tissue Repository is a veritable museum of disease, containing more than 2.5 million autopsy specimens dating back to the time of the Civil War.

Since 1918, the Spanish Lady has remained a weighty imponderable, a grave, ominous challenge to science. What made her so savage, so deadly? Her impudent disappearance seems the final insult. The greatest killer in human history vanished like an ephemeral will-o'-the-wisp, taking her secrets with her, dying with the dead. Even the isolation of the human influenza virus in 1933 did not help explain Spanish influenza's extraordinary ability to kill. The 1918 pandemic inspired the youthful discipline of virology to extraordinary progress, progress which would no doubt

219

have happened anyway, with or without the pandemic's conspicuous challenge. The identification of "filterable agents," the isolation and study of viruses, influenza research, and the
establishment of an international surveillance network to spare
millions flu's annual ills were inevitable. Even without a preoc-
cupation with Pfeiffer's bacillus, it is likely that some lucky, care-
less medical researcher would have left out a Petri dish of "cocci,"
and, like Dr. Alexander Fleming, returned to find the pesky
microorganisms devoured by penicillium mold. In 150 years,
medicine has enjoyed dazzling and abundant success. Still, the
pandemic remains lodged like a prickly thorn in the immense
body of accumulated medical knowledge. Rending science's most
triumphant era is the deadliest season of plague in the history of
human civilization: an irony so painful, so ominous that the pandemic has all but vanished from Earth's collective memory.

Who was the Spanish Lady? We now know she was an H1N1
virus, the first, deadly offspring of a new viral family. We suspect
a genetic mutation in late August allowed her to emerge in her
devastating "Second Act" as a true villain. But what, precisely,
made her so villainous? The question is not purely theoretical,
confined, like the epidemic itself, to the pages of history. Until
scientists understand what made Spanish influenza so lethal, we
remain vulnerable to a similar act of deadly caprice. The international surveillance network of the World Health Organization allows scientists to subtly track influenza's changes and to
man a line of defense through the manufacture of vaccines. But
in 1918, Spanish influenza hitched rides on Model Ts, trains,
and war ships and circumnavigated the globe in a matter of
weeks. Imagine the explosive swiftness of world-wide infection
in this age of jet travel. Influenza could engulf the world in a
matter of days, hardly allowing time enough to create and dis-
tribute a vaccine. An understanding of what made the 1918
virus so deadly is crucial. The secrets of Spanish influenza could

provide the critical tools needed to swiftly unlock the secrets of the next, inevitable pandemic.

In 1918, the Spanish Lady was everywhere. Soon she was nowhere. All over the world, medical researchers hunted her and viruses like her in labs. Others tried to find her, quite literally, in the grave. Perhaps, some scientists speculated, she might be resurrected from dead victims like Alaska's Eskimos, long-buried in the deep freeze of Earth's permafrost. A young Swedish pathologist, Dr. Johan V. Hultin, had this idea. Success was by no means certain. The natural contraction and expansion of the ground causes bodies in permafrost's active layer to drift upward over time and become vulnerable to summer thaw. Nevertheless, in 1950, Hultin, a doctoral student in microbiology at the State University of Iowa, proposed as his doctoral thesis an expedition to the northern coast of Alaska to exhume 1918 flu victims from permafrost. From a scientific standpoint, the mission was exhilarating. Perhaps it possessed a political urgency as well. The Cold War was escalating. Four hundred and fifty thousand Russians had died of Spanish influenza. What if America's Cold War enemy were to get the same idea as Hultin? Could a live 1918 virus be recovered from victims and used in biological warfare against the United States? Using mission records and weather charts, meticulously calculating annual deviations in the permafrost line, and cataloging the placement of bodies in mass graves, Hultin gauged where he was most likely to find success. He pinpointed three sites. Then, like scores of other doctoral students across the nation, Hultin applied for funding from the National Institutes of Health.

His idea had seemed a good one. But Hultin never heard back from the National Institutes of Health. Instead, according to Johan Hultin, the government simply co-opted his idea. In 1951, a secret U.S. military expedition was inaugurated to exhume influenza victims from Alaska's permafrost. Code-named Project

George, the three hundred thousand dollar mission was kept secret from the Russians and from a young Iowa doctoral student.
A serendipitous series of events led officials at the State University of Iowa to discover the government's plan; within 24 hours,
school officials had furnished Hultin with ten thousand dollars
and a ticket to Alaska. Hultin and his associates, Doctors Albert
McKee and Jack Layton, landed in Nome and quickly began ex-
cavating the first burial site. They discovered that a small creek
had changed course over time, rending the permafrost. The
corpses buried there would have decayed beyond scientific use-
fulness. The Iowans hired a bush pilot and flew off towards the
Seward Peninsula. Days later, massive Air Force transports
landed in Nome. Military personnel and enormous amounts of
heavy equipment were unloaded. The site was drilled and ex-
haustively excavated, but Project George turned up only bones.
The Iowa team had continued onto the village of Brevig Mission
(formerly Teller Mission). In one week in November 1918, 85
percent of Brevig Mission's inhabitants had perished. Victims
were exhumed. Tissue samples were excised from lungs, kidneys,
spleens, and brains. The specimens were carefully packed and returned to Iowa. They were comprehensively analyzed, but failed
to reveal any trace of live virus.

Nearly a half-century later, Dr. Jeffery K. Taubenberger, chief
of the division of molecular biology at the Armed Forces Institute of Pathology, was charged with the difficult task of recovering RNA virus from the severely decomposed flesh of dead
dolphins. Had the dolphins died of a measles-like virus or because of "red tide," as was originally believed? The challenge lay
not in the identification of the causative agent, but in the resurrection of virus from profoundly decayed tissue samples. Taubenberger and his team of scientists approached the dolphin project

with a combined expertise in pathology and molecular biology. To recover traces of virus from the pathologic specimen was the first challenge. To analyze the genetic material of the recovered strands of RNA was no less challenging. As Doctors Amy Krafft and Thomas Fanning and microbiologist Ann Reid painstakingly solved the problems posed by the dolphin project, Taubenberger wondered if these techniques might be put to another use. Would they allow the recovery of viruses from pathologic specimens housed in the National Tissue Repository, specimens taken from soldiers who had died of Spanish influenza? Would it be possible to find even *dead* viruses amid the shattered genetic landscapes of these tiny fragments of lung?

Taubenberger requisitioned three dozen pathologic specimens from the National Tissue Repository. He chose cases in which soldiers had died in the autumn of 1918 of massive pneumonia. The samples arrived—tiny scraps of lung tissue, preserved in formaldehyde, and embedded in small chunks of paraffin wax. For a year, Reid painstakingly scoured these flecks of lung for traces of an RNA virus. All the samples turned up negative. Then Krafft began analysis of the specimen from Private Roscoe Vaughn's lung. Luck was with her. There, amid the submicroscopic debris, were the minuscule remnants of an RNA virus.

In July 1996, the Spanish Lady was glimpsed for the first time. She took the lives of countless millions. Finally, one yielded her up.

In March 1997, Taubenberger and Reid published their findings in the journal *Science*. Catapulted into the international spotlight, Taubenberger found himself at the whirlwind center of the hunt for a killer virus. After nearly eighty years, the trail had suddenly become hot.

One man who greeted Taubenberger's work with special interest was a retired San Francisco pathologist. His name was Dr. Johan V. Hultin.

Hultin had read about Taubenberger's work in *Science*. From his excursion to Alaska in 1951, Hultin knew that no *live* virus had survived in Alaska's Eskimo victims. But now, in Taubenberger's lab, even a dead virus could be made to reveal its "genetic blueprint." In August 1997, Hultin asked Taubenberger if the A.F.I.P. team would analyze tissue samples from bodies exhumed from Alaska's permafrost if he were to get them. Taubenberger agreed. In this age of protracted, exhaustive planning and funding of scientific expeditions, Hultin told Taubenberger he could not leave "until next week." Days later, the seventy-three-year-old Hultin set off for Alaska, armed only with a sleeping roll, a camera, and two duffel bags full of tools and equipment.

In 1918, when influenza engulfed Alaska's Seward Peninsula, seventy-two of the eighty inhabitants of Teller Mission (now Brevig Mission) perished. The influenza victims were buried in a mass grave, marked with two large, wooden crosses. In August 1997, officials in Brevig Mission gave Hultin permission to exhume the dead. Four young men helped him dig. Hultin slept at night on the floor of the local school. The trench grew wider, longer, and deeper until it loomed twenty-seven feet long, six feet wide, and seven feet deep. Hutlin found bare skeletons, bones without soft tissue. Then he spied the well-preserved body of a woman. She was obese. Fat had protected her organs during decades of frost and thaw.

> I sat on a pail and looked at this woman. She was in a state of good preservation. Her lungs were good. I knew that this is where the virus would be.

Hultin named the woman "Lucy," after the skeleton which represents a critical prehistoric find. He took samples of her organs, packed them in preservative, and, to ensure the findings would not be lost, mailed four identical packages on four successive days, using Federal Express, United Parcel Service, and the U.S. Postal Service. He closed the grave site and crowned it with two wooden crosses, replicas of those used by missionaries in 1918. Hutlin made the crosses himself, in the woodshop of Brevig Mission's school.

A mere ten days later, Ann Reid discovered traces of the virus in Hultin's "Lucy." The virus matched the RNA found in Private Roscoe Vaughn's lung. Soon, a third match was made. The same virus was discovered in another specimen from the National Tissue Repository, a pathologic specimen taken from a thirty-year-old soldier, Private James Downs. Private Downs died of Spanish influenza in Camp Upton, New York, on September 26, 1918. The three samples were almost identical. Hultin's Alaskan find, drawn from a body in America's remotest province, had provided the necessary confirmation.

Scientists had found the Spanish Lady.

Small vials of a clear liquid line the shelf of a freezer, deep inside the Armed Forces Institute of Pathology. The liquid contains submicroscopic remnants of the 1918 virus. Reconstruction of the genetic structure of a dead virus is painfully slow work. Analysis of one of the virus's ten genes—the hemagglutinin gene—has been completed. Complete analysis of all the genes promises to help answer the critical question: what made Spanish influenza so lethal?

Preliminary analysis has revealed that Spanish influenza was a kind of H1N1 virus unlike any strain of human influenza identified in the past eighty years.

Spanish influenza most closely resembles "Swine Iowa 30," the pig flu isolated in 1930 by Dr. Richard Shope.

Nature's cunning is, of course, unparalleled. In a sublime act of natural mischief, Spanish influenza survives today in generation after changeable generation, in swine form, bringing the story full circle, or nearly full circle—forgetting only the bird.

The duck which flew south for winter.

We may never know where and when the fatal intersection(s) took place. Did the duck give influenza to a farmer? Did this happen in 1918, or years earlier? Did a pig prove the mixing vessel in which a savage duck-swine-human brew was concocted? Or did a feverish man, woman, or child give the virus to a pig in the fall of 1918, dooming swine to eternal cycles of annual disease?

We know the duck, the pig, and the man, woman, or child acted with the same profound innocence which inspires even nature's most savage acts. We now know that a crossroads, an intersection as chance and common as any bird passing overhead, casting a brief shadow across us, produced a complex, microscopic chain reaction which led to the wrenching human tragedy of Influenza 1918. In that season of plague, the tapestry of human life unraveled. William Maxwell lost his mother. Michael Wind entered the Hebrew Orphanage Asylum. Anna Milani lost her beloved Harry. Mary McCarthy lost her parents, Tessa and Roy. Woodrow Wilson, some historians suggest, lost hope. America's philosopher-president, at a critical moment in mankind's bloodiest century, lost heart. In a private moment of irrevocable loss, Katherine Anne Porter lost her lover, her one, "fine lieutenant." Porter's life, like the lives of so many others, was divided in two: before and after. That the pandemic seems banished to mankind's collective unconscious belies the experience of those who lived through it, who mended their lives, but who—in painful recollection—chronicle yet another generational cycle of human civilization, another parable of innocence and loss.

Selected Bibliography

The complete transcripts of the interviews conducted for the film, "Influenza 1918" (Producer: Robert Kenner; Writer: Ken Chowder) for *The American Experience* were invaluable. These transcripts included interviews with the following subjects:

John Deleno of New Haven, Connecticut.

Anna Milani, Columba Voltz, Susanna Turner, Harriet Ferrel, and Selma Epp of Philadelphia, Pennsylvania.

Lee Reay of Meadow, Utah.

Dan Tonkel of Goldsboro, North Carolina.

Books

Collier, Richard, *The Plague of the Spanish Lady*. Forge Village, MA: Murray Printing Co., 1974.

Crosby, Alfred, *Epidemic and Peace, 1918*. Westport, CT: Greenwood Press, 1976.

Hellemans, Alexander and Bryan Bunch, *The Timetables of Science*. Simon and Schuster, Inc., 1988.

Hoehling, A.A., *Disaster—Major American Tragedies*. New York: Hawthorne Books, Inc., 1973.

Hoehling, A.A., *The Great Epidemic—When the Spanish Influenza Struck*. Boston, Toronto: Little, Brown & Co., 1961.

Porter, Katherine Anne, *Pale Horse, Pale Rider and Other Stories*. New York: The New American Library of World Literature, Inc. (by arrangement with Harcourt, Brace & World, Inc.), 1936.

Porter, Roy, *Medicine: A History of Healing.* New York: Marlowe & Company; The Ivy Press, 1997.

Tucker, Spencer C., *The Great War 1914–18.* Bloomington: Indiana University Press, 1998.

Wilson, R. Jackson et. al, *The Pursuit of Liberty: A History of the American People.* Belmont, California: Wadsworth Publishing Company, 1990.

Articles

Fincher, Jack, "America's Deadly Rendezvous with the 'Spanish Lady.'" *Smithsonian.* Pp. 131–145.

Gladwell, Malcolm, "The Dead Zone." *The New Yorker,* Sept. 29, 1997. Pp. 52–65.

Henig, Robin Marante, "Flu Pandemic." *New York Times Magazine,* Nov. 29, 1992. Pp. 28–31, 55, 64, 66, 67.

Johnson, Judith R., "Kansas in the 'Grippe.' The Spanish Influenza Epidemic of 1918." *Kansas History,* Spring 1992. Pp. 44–55.

Kolata, Gina, "Lethal Virus Comes Out of Hiding." *New York Times (Science Times),* Feb. 24, 1998. Pp. C1, C5.

Larson, Erik, "The Flu Hunters." *Time Magazine.* Feb. 23, 1998. Pp. 55–64.

Persico, Joseph E., "The Great Swine Flu Epidemic of 1918." *American Heritage: The Magazine of History,* Vol. XXVII, No. 4, June, 1976. Pp. 28–31, 80–86.

Russell, Francis, "A Journal of the Plague: The 1918 Influenza." *The Yale Review.* Pp. 219–235.

Mayor Gilbert Tocktoo, "A Frozen Source of 1918 Flu Remnants." City of Brevig Mission, Alaska. Feb. 5, 1998.

The Armed Forces Institute of Pathology, "The A.F.I.P. Newsletter," Vol. 156, No. 2, April 1998.

Index

229

About the Author

A former Mirrielees Fellow in creative writing at Stanford University, LYNETTE IEZZONI is also a fiction writer, with a penchant for nineteenth-century medical history. She and writer Ken Chowder are developing a documentary film about nineteenth-century hysteria, an illness which affected an estimated two-thirds of all Victorian women. She is currently completing a novel, *Impasto*, the story of a painter who views her family's immigrant past and her own through the lens of art history. Iezzoni lives in northern California.

Photo Credits

The pictures in this book's photo gallery were provided courtesy of the following:

PAGE 1   Top: North Carolina Division of Archives, Raleigh.
Bottom: National Archives and Records Administration.

PAGE 2   Top: National Library of Medicine.
Bottom: National Archives and Records Administration.

PAGE 3   Iowa State University at Ames.

PAGE 4   National Archives and Records Administration.

PAGE 5   Top and bottom: U.S. Naval Historical Center.

PAGE 6   National Archives and Records Administration.

PAGE 7   Top: San Francisco Public Library.
Bottom: Otis Historical Archives, National Museum of Health and Medicine, Armed Forces Institute of Pathology.

PAGE 8   Otis Historical Archives, National Museum of Health and Medicine, Armed Forces Institute of Pathology.

PAGE 9   Top and bottom: National Archives and Records Administration.

PAGE 10   Top: RCC.
Bottom: Immigrant City Archives, Inc., Lawrence, MA.

PAGE 11   Top: National Archives.
Bottom: National Archives and Records Administration.

PAGE 12   Top and bottom: Photograph Archive, Utah State Historical Society.

PAGE 13   Top and bottom: National Archives and Records Administration.

PAGE 14   Top: California Historical Society. FN-30852.
Bottom: Colorado Historical Society.

PAGE 15   Oakland Public Library.

PAGE 16   California Historical Society. FN-24007.